T0259528

The Importance of the First Ray

Guest Editor

LAWRENCE A. FORD, DPM, FACFAS

CLINICS IN PODIATRIC MEDICINE AND SURGERY

www.podiatric.theclinics.com

Consulting Editor
THOMAS ZGONIS, DPM, FACFAS

July 2009 • Volume 26 • Number 3

SAUNDERS an imprint of ELSEVIER, Inc.

W.B. SAUNDERS COMPANY
A Division of Elsevier Inc.

1600 John F. Kennedy Boulevard • Suite 1800 • Philadelphia, Pennsylvania 19103-2899

http://www.theclinics.com

CLINICS IN PODIATRIC MEDICINE AND SURGERY Volume 26, Number 3
July 2009 ISSN 0891-8422, ISBN-13: 978-1-4377-1266-7, ISBN-10: 1-4377-1266-5

Editor: Patrick Manley
Developmental Editor: Donald Mumford

Clinics in Podiatric Medicine and Surgery (ISSN 0891-8422) is published quarterly by Elsevier Inc., 360 Park Avenue South, New York, NY 10010-1710. Months of publication are January, April, July, and October. Business and Editorial Offices: 1600 John F. Kennedy Blvd., Suite 1800, Philadelphia, PA 191023-2899. Customer Service Office: 6277 Sea Harbor Drive, Orlando, FL 32887-4800. Periodicals postage paid at New York, NY, and additional mailing offices. Subscription prices are $229.00 per year for US individuals, $360.00 per year for US institutions, $118.00 per year for US students and residents, $275.00 per year for Canadian individuals, $445.00 for Canadian institutions, $326.00 for international individuals, $445.00 per year for international institutions and $167.00 per year for Canadian and foreign students/residents. To receive student/resident rate, orders must be accompanied by name of affiliated institution, date of term, and the *signature* of program/residency coordinator on institution letterhead. Orders will be billed at individual rate until proof of status is received. Foreign air speed delivery is included in all *Clinics* subscription prices. All prices are subject to change without notice. POSTMASTER: Send address changes to *Clinics in Podiatric Medicine and Surgery*, Elsevier Periodicals Customer Service, 6277 Sea Harbor Drive, Orlando, FL 32887-4800. **Customer Service: 1-800-654-2452 (US). From outside of the US, call 314-453-7041. Fax: 314-453-5170. E-mail: JournalsCustomerService-usa@ elsevier.com (for print support); JournalsOnlineSupport-usa@elsevier.com (for online support).**

Reprints. For copies of 100 or more of articles in this publication, please contact the Commercial Reprints Department, Elsevier Inc., 360 Park Avenue South, New York, NY 10010-1710. Tel.: 212-633-3812; Fax: 212-462-1935; E-mail: reprints@elsevier.com.

Clinics in Podiatric Medicine and Surgery is covered in *MEDLINE/PubMed (Index Medicus) and EMBASE/Excerpta Medica.*

Printed and bound by CPI Group (UK) Ltd, Croydon, CR0 4YY

Transferred to Digital Print 2011

CLINICS IN PODIATRIC MEDICINE AND SURGERY

Contributors

CONSULTING EDITOR

THOMAS ZGONIS, DPM, FACFAS
Director, Podiatric Surgical Residency and Reconstructive Fellowship Programs;
Chief, Division of Podiatric Medicine and Surgery; Associate Professor, Department
of Orthopaedic Surgery, The University of Texas Health Science Center at San Antonio,
San Antonio, Texas

GUEST EDITOR

LAWRENCE A. FORD, DPM, FACFAS
Department of Orthopedics and Podiatric Surgery, The Kaiser Permanente Medical
Group; Program Director, Kaiser San Francisco Bay Area Foot and Ankle Residency
Program, Oakland, California

AUTHORS

NINA BABU-SPENCER, DPM
Kaiser San Francisco Bay Area Foot and Ankle Residency Program, Kaiser Foundation
Hospital, Oakland, California

RONALD BELCZYK, DPM
Fellow, Reconstructive Foot and Ankle Surgery and Clinical Instructor, Division of
Podiatric Medicine and Surgery, Department of Orthopaedic Surgery, University of Texas
Health Science Center at San Antonio, San Antonio, Texas

NEAL M. BLITZ, DPM, FACFAS
Chief of Foot Surgery, Department of Orthopaedic Surgery, Bronx-Lebanon Hospital
Center, Bronx, New York

PETER A. BLUME, DPM, FACFAS
Clinical Associate Professor, Department of Surgery, Yale School of Medicine;
Departments of Anesthesia, and Orthopaedics and Rehabilitation, Yale School of
Medicine, New Haven; Director, North American Center for Limb Preservation,
New Haven, Connecticut

PATRICK R. BURNS, DPM, FACFAS
Clinical Assistant Professor, Department of Orthopaedic Surgery, Division of Foot and
Ankle Surgery, University of Pittsburgh School of Medicine; Director, University
of Pittsburgh Medical Center Podiatric Residency Program, Pittsburgh, Pennsylvania

JEFFREY C. CHRISTENSEN, DPM
Director, Northwest Surgical Biomechanics Laboratory; Attending Podiatric Surgeon,
Department of Orthopedics, Division of Podiatric Surgery, Swedish Medical Center,
Seattle; Founder, Ankle and Foot Clinics Northwest, Everett, Washington

LAWRENCE A. FORD, DPM, FACFAS
Department of Orthopedics and Podiatric Surgery, The Kaiser Permanente Medical Group; Program Director, Kaiser San Francisco Bay Area Foot and Ankle Residency Program, Oakland, California

JORDAN P. GROSSMAN, DPM, FACFAS
Director, Podiatric Surgical Residency, Department of Surgery, Saint Vincent Charity Hospital, Cleveland, Ohio

ZACHARY M. HAAS, DPM
Albuquerque Associated Podiatrists, Albuquerque, New Mexico

SIGVARD T. HANSEN, Jr., MD
Professor, Department of Orthopaedics and Sports Medicine, University of Washington; Director, Foot and Ankle Institute, Harborview Medical Center, Seattle, Washington

GRAHAM A. HAMILTON, DPM, FACFAS
Department of Orthopedics and Podiatric Surgery, Kaiser Permanente Medical Center, Director of Education, Kaiser San Francisco Bay Area Foot and Ankle Residency Program, Antioch, California

CHRISTOPHER F. HYER, DPM, FACFAS
Director, Advanced Foot and Ankle Surgery Fellowship, Orthopedic Foot and Ankle Center, Westerville, Ohio

MEAGAN M. JENNINGS, DPM
Attending Podiatric Surgeon, Department of Orthopedics and Podiatry, Palo Alto Medical Foundation, Mountain View, California

THOMAS JORDAN, DPM
Chief Resident, San Francisco Bay Area Foot and Ankle Residency Program, San Francisco, California

ALISON M. JOSEPH, DPM
Podiatric Surgical Resident, University of Pittsburgh Medical Center, Pittsburgh, Pennsylvania

NICHOLAS J. LOWERY, DPM
Podiatric Surgical Resident, University of Pittsburgh Medical Center, Pittsburgh, Pennsylvania

SANDEEP PATEL, DPM
Department of Orthopedics and Podiatric Surgery, Kaiser Permanente Medical Center, Academic Director, Kaiser San Francisco Bay Area Foot and Ankle Residency Program, Antioch, California

SHANNON M. RUSH, DPM, FACFAS
Department of Orthopedics and Podiatric Surgery, The Palo Alto Medical Foundation, Camino Division, Mountain View, California

JOHN M. SCHUBERTH, DPM
Chief, Foot and Ankle Surgery, Department of Orthopedic Surgery, Kaiser Foundation Hospital, Site Director, Kaiser San Francisco Bay Area Foot and Ankle Residency Program, San Francisco, California

MATTHEW D. SORENSEN, DPM
Fellow, Advanced Foot and Ankle Surgery, Orthopedic Foot and Ankle Center, Westerville, Ohio

JOHN J. STAPLETON, DPM
Associate, Foot and Ankle Surgery, VSAS Orthopaedics, Allentown; Clinical Assistant Professor, Department of Surgery, Penn State College of Medicine, Hershey, Pennsylvania

THOMAS ZGONIS, DPM, FACFAS
Director, Podiatric Surgical Residency and Reconstructive Fellowship Programs; Chief, Division of Podiatric Medicine and Surgery; Associate Professor, Department of Orthopaedic Surgery, The University of Texas Health Science Center at San Antonio, San Antonio, Texas

Contents

For the past 100 years or so, the approach foot and ankle surgeons have taken too often has been to make compensating deformities or to do dysfunctional fusions. There is now a much improved understanding of the foot and attempt to restore normal anatomy, alignment, muscle balance, and function whenever possible. In a way, clinicians try to complete the evolutionary goal for the ideal foot for a biped. The first metatarsal is the key structure in this effort.

The first ray is the most important structure of the forefoot in its contribution to normal locomotion. Because first ray dysfunction is encountered in clinical practice with the development of hallux valgus, metatarsus primus varus, and hallux rigidus, there has been a belief that there is a mechanical basis for these conditions. Since publications in the 1930s, there has been significant research focused on the first ray. This article discusses the subtleties of normal and abnormal mechanics of the first ray to promote a better understanding for foot and ankle practitioners when treating these various disorders.

Medial column instability is a common and often complex condition that manifests as many associated clinical disorders. Progressive instability of the medial column usually is the result of equinus contracture, which leads to pathologic midfoot compensation. Lateral peritalar subluxation, posterior tibial tendon dysfunction, and functional impairment result. Stabilization of the medial column with naviculocuneiform arthrodesis addresses the pathology of the condition at the appropriate level and restores alignment to the arch and hindfoot.

The authors present a minimally invasive procedure for harvesting a split thickness skin graft (STSG) from the plantar surface of the foot. This is another option to consider for soft tissue reconstruction of diabetic foot wounds to help restore form and function and to prevent amputation. The authors do not recommend this technique for all soft tissue wounds of the toes and plantar aspect of the foot but believe it is a viable option for selected small diabetic foot wounds that may benefit from a STSG.

RELATED INTEREST

Clinics in Sports Medicine
Volume 27, Issue 2, Pages 247–338 (April 2008)
Foot and Ankle Injuries in Dance
Edited by J.G. Kennedy and C.W. Hodgkins

THE CLINICS ARE NOW AVAILABLE ONLINE!

Access your subscription at:
www.theclinics.com

Foreword

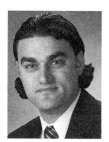

Thomas Zgonis, DPM, FACFAS
Consulting Editor

The intent of this issue is to emphasize the importance of understanding the normal and pathologic mechanics of the first ray. An outstanding group of foot and ankle experts present their interesting work related entirely to the first ray. This is an exciting issue in that a variety of foot conditions including but not limited to hallux valgus, hallux rigidus, metatarsalgia, pes planovalgus, and cavus deformities are described in detail by addressing the role of the first ray and medial column in each pathology.

Dr. Ford and his colleagues have done an extraordinary job of addressing the pathology associated with abnormalities about the first ray while simultaneously covering controversial issues in the scientific literature pertaining to the first ray. I am a strong advocate of understanding normal and pathologic mechanics about the first ray, especially when surgical management is influenced by the overall position and motion of the medial column of the foot. In addition, this issue also discusses the role of equinus and its effect on the first ray and foot pathology.

Finally, I would like to thank Dr. Hansen for his introduction and contribution to the *Clinics in Podiatric Medicine and Surgery.* I hope this issue will become a great tool to guide you when dealing with surgery of the first ray and addressing the mechanics and function of the foot.

Thomas Zgonis, DPM, FACFAS
Division of Podiatric Medicine and Surgery
Department of Orthopaedic Surgery
The University of Texas Health Science Center at San Antonio
7703 Floyd Curl Drive – MSC 7776
San Antonio, TX 78229

E-mail address: zgonis@uthscsa.edu

Clin Podiatr Med Surg 26 (2009) xv
doi:10.1016/j.cpm.2009.04.005
0891-8422/09/$ – see front matter © 2009 Elsevier Inc. All rights reserved.

Preface

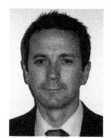

Lawrence A. Ford, DPM, FACFAS
Guest Editor

It is an honor to be able to bring together some of the brightest minds in foot and ankle surgery to share their passion and knowledge about the important role the first ray plays in the foot. Inherent to understanding foot pathology is a thorough understanding of normal and abnormal biomechanics of the foot. In pursuit of the reasons the foot fails and becomes pathologic, these surgeons believe that part of the answer lies in understanding the etiology.

The first ray is the major component of the medial column of the foot. Its dysfunction has far-reaching implications, from adult acquired flatfoot deformity to Charcot-Marie-Tooth Disease, central metatarsalgia, and, of course, hallux limitus and hallux valgus. A lot of attention has been given to these subjects in the literature, but there are still unanswered questions and there is so much more to learn. What defines the first ray and what is the best way to control it are points of controversy. Its power to create a cavus foot contrasted with its inability to support a flat foot has made it clear that there is also a continuum in between. The influence the first ray has on the foot that lies closer to the middle of this spectrum can be dramatic or subtle, but is nevertheless important. It is the purpose of this edition of *Clinics* to focus our attention on the first ray as an etiologic factor of deformity that must be addressed if the goal is to attempt to restore normal mechanics and function.

Lawrence A. Ford, DPM, FACFAS
Kaiser San Francisco Bay Area Foot and Ankle Residency Program
Department of Orthopedics and Podiatric Surgery
Kaiser Permanente Medical Center
Oakland, CA

E-mail address: lawrence.ford@kp.org

Clin Podiatr Med Surg 26 (2009) xvii
doi:10.1016/j.cpm.2009.04.004
0891-8422/09/$ – see front matter © 2009 Elsevier Inc. All rights reserved.

podiatric.theclinics.com

Introduction
The First Metatarsal: It's Importance in the Human Foot

Sigvard T. Hansen, Jr., MD

KEYWORDS

- Lapidus • Morton • Evolution • Atavistic traits
- Sagittal plane • Transverse plane
- Gastrocnemius equinus

My comments about the first metatarsal stem primarily from clinical observations over 45 years of interest in the foot and foot function. I had a specific interest in foot morphology and functional anatomy from even earlier time. As a second-year student in college, I took a course in comparative anatomy and soon thereafter became the student curator of the college's museum of natural history. In this role, I took student groups through the museum and explained the variations of color, stature, body conformation, beaks, claws, feet, and so forth as each bird or animal adapted to their niche in the environment. Being the son of a track coach, I was drawn early to observations of the leg and foot in humans and animals.

Gradually, over the first 10 years in practice dealing mostly with traumatology and pediatric and adult foot clinics, I realized that the standard treatments in both areas were not soundly based on functional anatomy and basic physiology and that they did not consider the possibility of evolutionary faults. It was also apparent that the best way to find better solutions to problems was by taking a very exacting history and physical examination of every patient seen in clinic, because there is no experimental animal that possesses a foot at all like the human foot. After doing this for several years, I came across a copy of Morton's book[1] in which many ideas were clearly laid out and pathophysiology described that closely paralleled my developing ideas. I had already adopted the Lapidus procedure in young patients as a solution to adolescent bunion problems. I had tried the standard McBride and Silver procedures and even the Keller procedure for older people, popular in the 1960s, and they clearly were not effective in adolescents.

The results in these patients were already markedly improved when Morton's book became my guide to developing treatments and protocols for foot and ankle reconstruction. Careful observation revealed that a high percentage of foot problems in

Harborview Medical Center, 6th Floor, East Clinic, Box 359799, 325 Ninth Avenue, Seattle, WA 98104, USA
E-mail address: hansetmd@u.washington.edu

Clin Podiatr Med Surg 26 (2009) 351–354
doi:10.1016/j.cpm.2009.03.012
0891-8422/09/$ – see front matter © 2009 Elsevier Inc. All rights reserved.

adults were associated with, if not caused by, gastrocnemius equinus. This was not new information, but it was controversial. I had taken a 6-month job as a senior house officer at Sheffield Children's Hospital in Sheffield, England, in 1970 where I did a fellowship in pediatric neuromuscular orthopedics. I learned to do a thorough and complete examination of all muscles in the foot as part of defining neurologic levels in patients with meningomyelocele, polio, cerebral palsy (CP), Charcot-Marie-Tooth disease, clubfoot, and so forth.

If one does this with a completely open mind, it can produce science, defined as knowledge of foot and ankle function and pathology, and lead to treatment protocols based on causation. This is very important, especially for those who choose to believe only those things proved by a truly scientific method. Personally, I trust my clinical observations over and above "studies." In reality, there is a constant interplay of bony structures, ligaments, muscle balance, and neurologic control all modulated by what has happened in the past. Other factors include patients' individual personalities, lifestyle, and so forth. No laboratory study can mimic the full range of interactions among all these tissues and the nervous system even though certain aspects of things can be studied in a very controlled way.

In reviewing my clinical observations, especially the results of my treatment protocols based on cause and effect relationships, I see the first metatarsal as one of the key structures necessary to understand completely how to manage foot problems. The foot's stability and position in the sagittal plane determines whether a patient has a cavus, plantar grade, or pronated foot. The first metatarsal normally bears about a third of the weight across the forefoot.[2] The weight in the forefoot is ideally borne relatively equally between the two sesamoids and each of the four lesser metatarsal heads.

In the transverse plane, spreading or splaying of the first metatarsal from its normal alignment beside the second metatarsal increases the probability of the so-called "bunion," an inadequate term describing metatarsus primus varus and secondarily hallux valgus.

By 1975, having read all the theories and having tried many of the operations published at the time with varying success, I read Lapidus' paper.[3] The theory of hypermobility in the first ray appealed to me, but not the cat-gut fixation. I had become proficient by that time with Arbeitsgemeinschaft Fur Osteosynthesefragen (AO) fixation through trauma work and began performing the Lapidus procedure using compression screw fixation instead of soft fixation. The Lapidus procedure is associated with a very rational capsulorrhaphy at the metatarsophalangeal joint and immediately it showed much more reliable results than the modified McBride and Silver procedures that we were performing in patients in their mid and late teens (with epiphyses closed usually). Early on, we were not looking for or treating the gastrocnemius equinus that I now believe is commonly present and did not do gastroc slides on our younger patients. Even so, the results were very good. Somewhat later, we began performing Strayer procedures, and then because of scarring we switched to percutaneous tendo-Achilles lengthening. Later still, we went back to the gastroc slide on the theory that there is no rationale for lengthening the soleus, which is rarely part of the contracture in these cases.

In older patients we saw associated claw toes with extensor dominance, metatarsalgia, and so forth and added Girdlestone procedures and extensor lengthening, and later extensor substitution or transfer by moving the extensor digitorum longus to the peroneus tertius and motoring the distal long extensors with the short extensors. Simple extensor lengthening often resulted in scarring down and holding the toes contracted in extension.

Complete attention to all of the deformities and all the predisposing atavistic traits has the potential to provide outstanding results both in the short and long term. The problem is that it can be a very demanding surgical procedure and also quite tedious and time-consuming if the entire adjunctive and toe tendon transfers are performed. It does not fit the common criteria for a "good" procedure if that is construed to be quick and easy and covered by insurance. It is clearly based on a thorough understanding of what the first ray particularly and what the foot in general should be like in a normal situation and trying to recreate that by solving causative or aggravating problems and the secondary pathology that developed.

From the standpoint of comparative anatomy, and with a nod to evolution, the human foot is strongly characterized and its function is maximized by the first metatarsal. In other animals, particularly four-legged animals that rely on speed, the first metatarsal is vestigial and the middle metatarsals are predominant. Their foot function occurs at the end of the metatarsals or phalanges rather than on a flat foot from the calcaneus forward. In our closer relatives the anthropoids (apes, chimpanzees, bonobos, and even monkeys) the first metatarsal is very important but is used primarily as an opposable digit for grasping and is a weight-bearing structure only part time on flat surfaces, but it is the most dominant digit.

The bipedal human ability to balance on a single limb seems to be closely related to the development and evolution of the first metatarsal into a very stable structure. The first metatarsal is part of the arch on the medial side of the foot, which protects the entry of the extrinsic tendons and the neurovascular structures to the more distal foot, and its controlling musculature and ligamentous stability are essential for balancing on one limb.

It is of interest that the first metatarsal has much more and different muscle attachments than the other metatarsals and a much broader and stronger toe which, like the thumb, has two phalanges rather than three. The two sesamoids in the short flexor tendons are of similar size and of the same weight-bearing distribution as the lesser metatarsal heads. This means that two of the six weight-bearing points in the foot and nearly a third of the body's weight are borne on the front of the foot going into the first metatarsal.

Two powerful extrinsic muscles, the long peroneal and the tibialis anterior, attach to the inferior surface of the proximal end of the metatarsal. The long peroneal plantar flexes and supinates the first metatarsal and forefoot and the anterior tibialis dorsiflexes and pronates the first metatarsal and forefoot. This terminology is confusing in that when the forefoot is supinated, the hindfoot is allowed to pronate and vice versa.

The powerful intrinsic short flexors of the great toe arrive from the first metatarsal near the base and attach to the sesamoids in the proximal phalanges. The long extrinsics going to the great toe are connected primarily only to the great toe. The extensor hallucis longus is a separate muscle from the extensor digitorum longus. It dorsiflexes the great toe at the interphalangeal joint while the extensor digitorum longus dorsiflexes the remainder of the lesser toes through the distal phalangeal joints. The short extensors dorsiflex at the metatarsophalangeal joints. Likewise, the flexor hallucis longus primarily flexes only the great toe through the interphalangeal joint and is a totally separate muscle from the flexor digitorum longus, which goes to all of the lesser toes. A surgically important fact, however, is that the flexor hallucis longus almost always sends a slip of the long flexor to the second toe and frequently to the third toe.

Finally, the first tarsometatarsal joint is normally quite stable even though it has one less ligament than the bases of the second and third metatarsals, which are indeed very stable in the normal individual. Morton demonstrated that the first tarsometatarsal joint alone or together with the first intercuneiform joint and naviculocuneiform joints can be excessively mobile, possibly reflecting the different evolution in the apes that leaves the first ray mobile enough to be opposable to the remaining metatarsals and toes. This is detrimental to the normal function of the human first metatarsal, which requires stability for optimal function. Again, Morton has shown that with excessive dorsal mobility the first metatarsal transfers weight laterally. When this occurs, the foot pronates and has much less effective propulsion. The second or other lesser metatarsals may develop overload symptoms with findings that include callousing and even keratosis under the head, synovitis, and synovitic capsular damage in the metatarsophalangeal joints, and subluxation or dislocation. Over the long term, osseous hypertrophy of the second metatarsal may occur sometimes causing second metatarsal stress fractures. Proximal second or second and third tarsometatarsal overload can cause synovitis and eventual arthritis and sometimes collapse and deformity in the forefoot. All these pathologic tendencies are made worse in patients who are overweight or those who have excessive gastrocnemius tone or function.[4]

The medial column is composed of the talus, navicular, first cuneiform, and first metatarsal. It normally has a moderately arched configuration. The lateral column is composed of the calcaneus, cuboid, and fourth and fifth metatarsals and is moderately flat, at least without any discernible arch in the normal situation.

Dilwyn Evans likely introduced the concept that the normal foot and foot function depend on the correct relationship of the medial and lateral columns. In effect, the medial and lateral sides of the foot adjust the position of the forefoot and midfoot in relation to the hindfoot.

Hindfoot refers to the talus and calcaneus, the midfoot to the navicular and cuboid and first, second, and third cuneiforms. The forefoot consists of the metatarsals and phalanges. The position of the first metatarsal in the transverse and sagittal planes is critical to the alignment of the whole mechanism and is dependent on the stability of the tarsometatarsal joint. One should keep in mind that many other features including the plantar fascia, the long and short plantar ligaments, and intrinsic and extrinsic tendon balance are also important factors.[4]

SUMMARY

For the past 100 years or so, the approach foot and ankle surgeons have taken too often has been to make compensating deformities or to do dysfunctional fusions. There is now a much improved understanding of the foot and attempt to restore normal anatomy, alignment, muscle balance, and function whenever possible. In a way, the attempt is to complete the evolutionary goal for the ideal foot for a biped. The first metatarsal is the key structure in this effort.

REFERENCES

1. Morton DJ. The human foot. Columbia University Press; 1935.
2. Hughes J, Clark P, Linge K, et al. A comparison of two studies of the pressure distribution under the feet of normal subjects using different equipment. Foot Ankle 1993;14(9):514–9.
3. Lapidus PW. Operative correction of the metatarsis primus varus in hallux valgus. In: Surg Gynecol Obstet 1934;58:183–91.
4. Johnson CH, Christensen JC. Biomechanics of the first ray part V: the effect of equinus deformity: a 3-dimensional kinematic study on a cadaver model. J Foot Ankle Surg 2005;44(2):114–20.

Normal and Abnormal Function of the First Ray

Jeffrey C. Christensen, DPM[a,b,c,*], Meagan M. Jennings, DPM[d]

KEYWORDS

- First ray hypermobility • First ray insufficiency • Hallux valgus
- Hallux limitus • Biomechanics

Functionally, the foot and leg, with multiple moving segments and variable loads coupled with striking anatomic variability, create a locomotive complexity that makes understanding biomechanical relationships a challenge. It is well known from pressure analysis studies that the load bearing of the forefoot is three times that of the hindfoot.[1] The first ray (FR), comprised of the first metatarsal and medial cuneiform,[2,3] is arguably the most dominant mechanical structure of the forefoot. As a result, its proper function is critical; however, it is susceptible to a variety of pathomechanical conditions. Duchenne[4] recognized that the functional position of the FR is dependent on agonist-antagonist muscle balance of the peroneus longus (PL), tibialis anterior, and tibialis posterior. Yet, more than 140 years later, there still is significant confusion and clinical ambiguity in the literature regarding normal and abnormal FR mechanics. At the pinnacle of controversy is FR hypermobility, which has been used to characterize FR excursion that is greater than normal. Although there is general consensus that the condition exists, the term lacks precise definition and clear understanding among foot and ankle specialists. Being mindful of some of these pervasive controversies that exist in the literature, the authors focus on a conceptual approach to advance mechanical concepts of the FR that can be best supported by the accumulated evidence, hopefully clarifying some of these misconceptions.

It was the works of Morton and Lapidus that ignited modern controversies concerning FR dysfunction. Conditions of atavistic traits,[5,6] dorsal first metatarsal segment hypermobility,[7–9] and transverse instability were reported.[5] It is established that the

[a] Northwest Surgical Biomechanics Laboratory, Swedish Medical Center-Cherry Hill Campus, 500-17th Avenue, Seattle, WA 98122, USA
[b] Division of Podiatric Surgery, Department of Orthopedics, Swedish Medical Center, Seattle, WA, USA
[c] Ankle & Foot Clinics Northwest, 3131 Nassau Street, Suite 101, Everett, WA 98201, USA
[d] Department of Orthopedics and Podiatry, Palo Alto Medical Foundation, 701 East. El Camino Real, Mountain View, CA 94040, USA
* Corresponding author. Division of Podiatric Surgery, Department of Orthopedics, Swedish Medical Center, Seattle, WA.
E-mail address: jccdpm@gmail.com (J.C. Christensen).

Clin Podiatr Med Surg 26 (2009) 355–371
doi:10.1016/j.cpm.2009.03.004
0891-8422/09/$ – see front matter © 2009 Elsevier Inc. All rights reserved.

podiatric.theclinics.com

FR is essential for transmission of weight-bearing forces and maintaining arch stability in midstance and propulsive phases of gait (**Fig. 1**). To accomplish this, the FR requires a delicate balance of ligamentous and muscle support to maintain functional segmental alignment. The static stability comes from the intermetatarsal, plantar metatarsocuneiform, and interosseous ligaments and the medial fibers of the central band of the plantar fascia.[10–12] Dynamic and static stabilization of the FR is essential during locomotion to prepare the foot for resupination via the windlass mechanism.[3,13] The human foot functions as a lever going into propulsion and uses the hallux windlass to impart stability to the FR. Malfunction of the FR and windlass mechanism affect efficient load transmission to the forefoot and subject adjacent pedal structures to increased load stresses and possible mechanical breakdown.

MUSCULAR STABILIZERS

Dynamic stabilizers are probably the least understood factor when reviewing the normal and abnormal mechanics of the forefoot. Dynamic stabilizers of the FR and medial arch include primarily the posterior tibial (PT), PL, flexor hallucis brevis (FHB), and flexor hallucis longus (FHL).[11,14] When the PL contracts in closed kinetic chain, there is a triplane moment applied to the FR in the direction of eversion, plantarflexion, and abduction.[15] The dorsal to plantar height of the medial cuneiform is nearly twice the size of the remaining cuneiforms. This anatomic design combined with the extreme plantar insertion of the PL provides a significant torsional leverage against the intermediate cuneiform (**Fig. 2**). The eversion moment combined with the wedge shape of the osseous segments provides a locking mechanism via a closed packed position of the medial and intermediate cuneiforms.[15,16] This has a stabilizing role and can control sagittal plane excursion independent to any existing plantarflexory moment. Normally the course of the PL across the plantar arch follows an inclined path from the pulley of the cuboid to its insertion. This provides mechanical advantage to the PL to help counter midstance ground reactive loads on the FR. The tendon inclination across the arch is reduced with medial arch depression making the plantarflexory pull less efficient with a pronated foot architecture. In a lesser-known attribute, the FHL and FDL during gait reduce the magnitude of dorsal strain of the metatarsals incurred from ground reactive forces.[17,18] This function probably plays a more important role in the second metatarsal, because it is more susceptible to dorsal strain, especially when there is FR dysfunction. Sharkey and colleagues[17] demonstrated in their elaborate laboratory study that FHL function also reduces dorsal but simultaneously increases medial second metatarsal strain. Intrinsic muscles

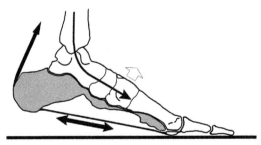

Fig. 1. Diagram depicts a rigid beam of the medial column as a function of the windlass mechanism and a stable FR. Load can pass through the FR as the entire forefoot shares in load transmission.

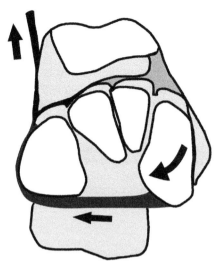

Fig. 2. Diagram of cross section through the midfoot along with the distal course of the PL. Note the torsional lever arm of the medial cuneiform with the action of the PL and the wedge shape of the intermediate cuneiform that can control dorsal migration of the FR.

contract in late midstance and into propulsion.[19] FHB is an important stabilizer of the hallux during gait and helps to transfer loads anteriorly to the hallux.

THE ROLE OF THE WINDLASS MECHANISM

The plantar fascia is a durable structure that receives combined load from body weight and from generated Achilles tension during midstance phase of gait.[20–22] It also provides significant arch-supporting function.[14,23] The forces generated in the plantar fascia gradually increase during midstance and peak in late stance.[21] The concept of the windlass effect was first advanced by Hicks.[13] It is the passive tensioning of the plantar fascia that occurs during gait when the foot enters propulsive phase. The windlass is most powerful at the first metatarsophalangeal joint (MTPJ) due to the leverage generated through the sesamoids and the larger arc of curvature of the first metatarsal head.[13] During heel lift, the hallux and lesser toes remain purchased on the ground as the foot rises and rotates over the fixed digits. The resultant dorsiflexion increases tension of the plantar fascia and shortens its working distance inducing: increased arch height, metatarsal plantarflexion, arch joint compression/stabilization, and calcaneal inversion.[13,20,24] The sesamoids can be seen moving anterior to the metatarsal head. As the windlass engages in propulsion, the first metatarsal will plantarflex and induce increased plantar pressures while simultaneously the second metatarsal pressures will decrease.[25]

The windlass helps propel the body on its release at the point of push off,[26] but it also works in reverse with forefoot loading as the body load flattens the arch and unwinds the windlass allowing the toes to plant and grip the ground.[13] Sectioning the plantar aponeurosis negates the windlass[20,27] and shifts static load from the digits to the metatarsal heads.[21,28]

FIRST RAY FUNCTION IN GAIT

In normal gait there is a smooth and rapid transition of load from the heel to the forefoot.[1] The precise movements of the osseous segments of the foot historically have been only approximations because of limitations of tracking individual bones in space. Gait systems with skin-mounted sensors have significant errors when compared with true osseous kinematic motion.[29] Lundgren and colleagues tracked individual osseous movements of the foot segments in vivo in 6 normal volunteers during walking. To improve accuracy, the investigators used sensors attached directly to Kirschner wires surgically placed in the bone segments. The results revealed that the majority of motion at the FR occurs at the naviculocuneiform joint (sagittal 11.5° [SD = 1.8°], frontal 10.4° [SD = 6.3°], and transverse 6.2° [SD = 4.2°]) with approximately 50% less motion at the first metatarsocuneiform joint (sagittal 5.3° [SD = 2.0°], frontal 5.4° [SD = 1.0°], and transverse 6.1° [SD = 1.1°]).[30]

The metatarsal heads bear load for approximately 80% of stance phase of gait.[31] There are, however, variable metatarsal loading patterns that are seen between the first and second rays.[32–37] It has been observed that the ratio of peak pressures between the first and second metatarsal heads correlate with relative protrusion of the metatarsal segments.[32,34]

FIRST RAY INSUFFICIENCY

FR insufficiency is best described as a syndrome: a collection of signs and symptoms that present clinically caused by a dynamic imbalance between the first and second metatarsal segments to transmit body weight. FR insufficiency can be caused by FR hypermobility, segmental length disorders, or structural malalignments. Independent to underlying etiology, the clinical presentation involves dysfunctional load transfer capacity of the first metatarsal with overload compensation of the lesser metatarsals namely the second and occasionally the third metatarsal segments.

Signs and symptoms of FR insufficiency include increased pronation, diffuse plantar callus formation at second or third metatarsal head, metatarsalgia, plantar second metatarsal base tenderness, relative widening of second metatarsal shaft and cortical thickening, absence of first metatarsal plantar callus formation, subluxation/dislocation second MTPJ, and lesser metatarsal stress fractures.[7,8,38–40] The authors stress the importance of understanding that FR hypermobility can cause FR insufficiency; however, because there are other determinants (eg, the windlass mechanism) that can contribute to FR stability in gait, the presence of FR hypermobility alone does not prohibit the FR in performing its normal function of load transmission in the right setting.

SHORT FIRST METATARSAL SEGMENT

Morton introduced the condition of "metatarsus ataviscus" (congenital short first metatarsal) in 1927 as a distinct clinical entity, which was later coined, "Morton's foot."[6] He related foot dysfunction to this short metatarsal segment, which he believed caused increased pronation to allow the first metatarsal to engage the ground and thus compensatory load transmission diverting to the second ray.[8] In midstance a subtle amount of shortness easily can be compensated for by the action of PL to increase metatarsal declination and through the windlass mechanism. The critical level of shortness in an individual depends on foot type, angle of gait, body weight, and Achilles tightness among other factors. In these critical levels of shortening, the first metatarsal may be able to purchase the ground in midstance; however, FR insufficiency is seen in propulsion where the first metatarsal is incapable of sustaining load transfer due to the forward extension of the second metatarsal segment. Symptoms of metatarsalgia can be elicited, but even though the condition is considered congenital, the clinical expression of the disorder usually is in adult life (**Fig. 3**). Morton's analysis of the mechanical deficiencies behind a short first metatarsal segment seems to have

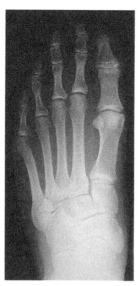

Fig. 3. Case example of congenital short first metatarsal. The first metatarsal was 15 mm shorter than the second. The patient participated in college athletics and was only mildly symptomatic. He did not become severely symptomatic until his early 30s, several years after college graduation. He developed severe metatarsalgia subsecond metatarsal.

stood the test of time. This is especially true in patients who have severe iatrogenic shortening of the first metatarsal (**Fig. 4**).

In patients who have a short first metatarsal segment, Morton also described clinical tenderness at the second metatarsal base (**Fig. 5**).[6] This clinical effect was affirmed

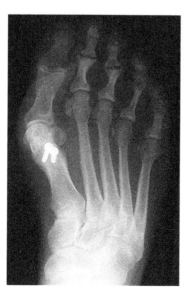

Fig. 4. Iatrogenic first metatarsal shortening and malunion postbunionectomy; note compensatory thickening of second and third metatarsals. Clinically the patient exhibited severe metatarsalgia symptoms subsecond metatarsal.

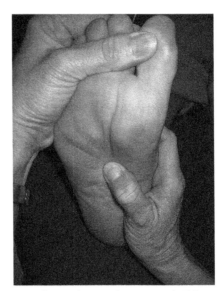

Fig. 5. Palpation maneuver at base of second metatarsal. This can be indicative of lesser metatarsal overload from FR insufficiency.

and further advanced by Davitt and colleagues,[41] who associated a short first metatarsal with second metatarsal base arthrosis (**Fig. 6**). In their series, the study group's second metatarsal functional length was 18.6% greater than the first metatarsal as compared with 4.1% in the control group. This is a logical relationship, because the base of the second metatarsal is approximately only one half the height of the first metatarsal, and the second metatarsocuneiform joint does not have a corresponding

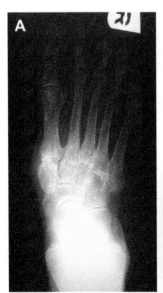
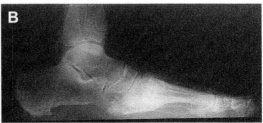

Fig. 6. Radiographic example of Morton's foot with midfoot arthrosis. The patient had no history of midfoot trauma. (*A*) AP view. (*B*) Lateral view.

plantar ligament.[11] Thus, the second metatarsal is ill prepared to endure increased stresses over long periods of time.

Morton was the first to observe the second metatarsal cortical thickening and shaft widening as compensation for mechanical deficiencies of the FR (**Fig. 7**). He used a formula to take into account changes in metatarsal width, cortical thickness, and relative metatarsal structure of adjacent lesser metatarsals.[8] The concept of second metatarsal hypertrophy in FR hypermobility has been challenged.[42–44] Grebing and Coughlin[43] compared second metatarsal radiographic characteristics in 4 diagnostic groups (43 patients each): controls (asymptomatic feet), hallux valdus, hallux rigidus, and neuroma. They used Morton's same formula and concluded that there was no significant difference between groups regarding hypertrophy of the second meta-tarsal. They did not match relative metatarsal length with their treatment groups and controls, however. The control group had the greatest incidence of short first meta-tarsal (30% as compared with 5% for hallux valgus and 14% for hallux rigidus using arc method of measurement). The control group appeared to have second metatarsal cortical thickening possibly from the higher incidence of short first metatarsal. Other articles studied only changes in width and cortical thickening of the second metatarsal and tried to correlate thickness with dorsal mobility of the FR; they found significant correlation, however, relative metatarsal length was not measured.[42,44] It is clear that that further research is needed in this area.

FIRST RAY HYPERMOBILITY

A pronatory moment of the foot can overload the medial column and increase loads crossing the FR.[45,46] The FR in this setting is susceptible to developing well-recog-nized pathomechanical conditions, including metatarsus primus varus, metatarsus primus elevatus, and overload symptoms affecting the second metatarsal segment,

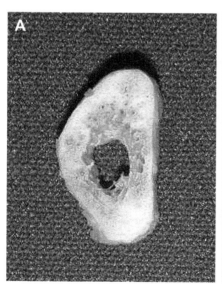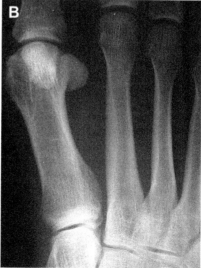

Fig. 7. (*A*) Second metatarsal midshaft specimen from a Morton's foot removed during a second metatarsal shortening procedure. Note the marked dorsal and plantar thickening. (*B*) Radiograph of second metatarsal thickening from mild hallux valgus deformity and short first metatarsal.

which all can be attributed to dorsal FR hypermobility. Morton first described the concept of hypermobility without hallux valgus deformity in 1928[7]:

> Hypermobility of the first metatarsal bone would hardly constitute a factor in foot trouble if the increased arch of motion were located entirely in the plantar direction; the fault lies in the increase of dorsal movement, or hyperextension, of the first metatarsal bone, whereby the normal stability of the inner border of the foot becomes reduced or lost.
>
>   When body-weight is imposed upon a foot, the slack of the plantar ligaments must be taken up before the load is actually supported. In a foot of the type under consideration, the plantar structure attached to the four outer metatarsal bones becomes taut, while the inner pillar of the foot is still a lax and yielding member. Thus, the second metatarsal bone is compelled to bear the brunt of the load, or yielding to some degree, to share it with the third.

Since Morton's insights into the concept of dorsal hypermobility, clinicians have focused on manual assessment of static excursion between the first and second metatarsal segments in the sagittal plane, by moving the FR until resistance is met and using the level of the second metatarsal plantarly as a neutral reference.[3,8] The concept of a hypermobile first metatarsal segment generally has been accepted especially in severe cases; however, there is controversy in defining milder forms of the condition and its clinical expression. There has been great interest in accurately quantitating static FR excursion in attempt to better define hypermobility. Methodology and patient selection have been variable.[24,38,42,44,47–61]

The end product of sagittal first metatarsal displacement is the aggregative ligamentous, plantar fascial, and tendinous constraints crossing collective segmental articulations of first MTPJ and intercuneiform, first metatarsocuneiform, intermetatarsal, naviculocuneiform, and talonavicular joints. The investigations (cited above) describe only the end product of motion and not the relative joint contribution because the technique used cannot ascertain the motion origin. Klaue and colleagues[57] measured the displacement at the neck and the base of the metatarsal to get an estimate of the center of rotation in his series and suggested that the origin of the motion was at the metatarsocuneiform joint. This, however, contrasts with Roling and colleagues,[59] who determined that the naviculocuneiform was the major contributor to FR motion.

The hypermobile FR that becomes clinically problematic exhibits dysfunction during late midstance and early propulsion where the windlass mechanism normally engages, the stabilizing muscles are contracting, and the velocity of load transfer is the greatest. If the distal first metatarsal segment is still able to elevate as the windlass engages, then the foot pronates and load shifts laterally to the lesser metatarsals. The FR also can lack hypermobility on clinical examination and still be functionally insufficient if the windlass mechanism is compromised.

The relationship of FR static mobility and dynamic FR sagittal motion during gait has been examined previously.[62] The study concludes FR static mobility on clinical examination is a poor predictor of abnormal first metatarsal function in gait. Windlass function needs to be assessed with hypermobility to obtain a more accurate picture in predicting FR insufficiency.

THE WINDLASS ACTIVATION TEST

Rush and colleagues[23] was the first investigation to test the concept of engaging the windlass when evaluating FR competency. This theory uses windlass engagement during the evaluation of FR sagittal excursion; Christensen described testing the windlass function in a clinical setting that can better predict the FR stability during propulsion.[24,63,64] In a patient who has had a previous Keller bunionectomy or overlengthening from plantar fascia release, dorsiflexion of the hallux has minimal effect in imparting stability to the FR. To the contrary, the windlass does not engage and FR dorsal excursion is unaffected with hallux position (**Fig. 8**).

HALLUX VALGUS PATHOMECHANICS

There is increased FR sagittal and transverse mobility associated with hallux valgus deformity that appears as continuum of severity depending on the degree of metatarsus primus varus deformity. Hallux valgus with metatarsus primus varus can circumvent the direct lever effects of the windlass.[24] The deviated hallux has an effectively shorter lever arm with a net vector force that subsequently leads to first metatarsal escape, a transverse migration of the first metatarsal head medially. This is a mechanical dampening effect with a less efficient hallux lever causing delay of windlass engagement. The windlass tension and FHB pull with the deviated hallux can cause the metatarsal to splay farther into varus and make the first metatarsal segment incompetent to share equal load with the second metatarsal segment. End-stage hallux valgus ultimately can lead to increased pronation and breakdown of the plantar ligaments, which can impair various structures along the medial column and can compromise effective gait (**Fig. 9**).

Transverse instability of the FR also has been demonstrated in hallux valgus.[5,43,50,65–68] This has been quantified radiographically in reduction and provocation of the intermetatarsal angle.[38,66,68–70] Weber and colleagues[68] suggested that an outward splaying of the metatarsal may be more effective in testing the level of transverse instability than by compressing the metatarsals.

It has been shown, in cadaver models and in patients who have hallux valgus and an increased intermetatarsal angle, that there is an increase in sagittal FR static displacement.[24,48,49,53] This sagittal hypermobility is largely dependent on FR malposition; thus, with segmental realignment, the sagittal plane FR mobility returns to normal and the windlass becomes more efficient.

Hallux valgus deformity also seems to have an impact on the frontal plane mechanics of the FR. When the FR is inverted, there is significantly greater sagittal

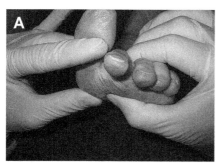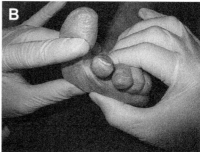

Fig. 8. Case example of patient who had severe subsecond metatarsalgia after plantar fascia release and overlengthening. There is no evidence of FR hypermobility and the metatarsals I and II are of equal length and declination. The windlass activation test was performed and revealed there was persistent FR mobility with the windlass engaged explaining the metatarsalgia. Lack of dynamic load sharing of the first and second metatarsals was confirmed with pedobarographic testing. (*A*) Starting position after windlass activation. (*B*) FR elevates with manual testing.

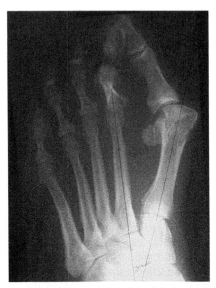

Fig. 9. Radiograph end stage hallux valgus deformity with dorsal dislocated second toe from chronic lesser metatarsal overload and first metatarsocuneiform arthrosis.

mobility compared with an everted FR position.[15,16] It is unclear how the architecture of hallux valgus and metatarsus primus varus affects this mechanism; however, inter-cuneiform widening often is seen in advanced metatarsus primus varus.

SURGICAL EFFECTS IN HALLUX VALGUS SURGERY

Iatrogenically induced FR insufficiency from ablative FR procedures (ie, implant and resection arthroplasty) results in a loss of sesamoid function and the ability to stabilize the FR via the windlass mechanism (**Fig. 10**).[71,72] The ability of the foot to engage the windlass mechanism is dependent on a fully corrected FR, which maintains functional

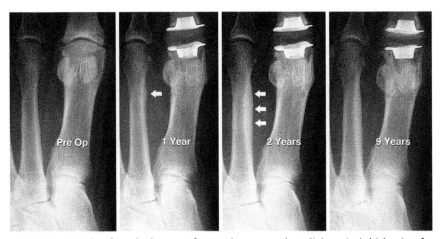

Fig. 10. Case example of gradual onset of second metatarsal medial cortical thickening from iatrogenic FR insufficiency after placement of total silicone implant.

length and realigns the metatarsal with the sesamoid apparatus and hallux. Any process that leads to altered length-tension relationship of this mechanism induces lesser metatarsal overload. This is classically seen after Keller bunionectomy with the development of stress fractures postoperatively[73,74] but can occur with any bunionectomy that shortens or elevates the first metatarsal (**Fig. 11**).[5,75,76] Direct evidence of second metatarsal overload has been measured dynamically in postbunionectomy patients who have crescentic osteotomy of the first metatarsal base where first metatarsal elevation was observed.[76]

HALLUX LIMITUS/RIGIDUS PATHOMECHANICS

There seems to be a continuum of pathology with a rectus hallux associated with feet that exhibit an increased pronation moment with medial column overload. This begins with a condition referred to a functional hallux limitus where there is significant resistance to hallux dorsiflexion in early propulsion, but in open kinetic chain there is no restriction of first MTPJ motion. Although the reverse windlass forces the hallux to plantarflex and purchase the ground, if the windlass engages to rapidly, then the proximal phalanx has reduced capacity to induce FR plantarflexion. This has a jamming effect on the joint. As the pathology worsens, there is progressive joint degeneration initially along the dorsal half of the MTPJ with focal erosions at the metatarsal head and early dorsal metatarsal spurring.[77,78] With further progression, the head of the metatarsal flattens and medial and lateral osteophytes develop as the dorsal osteophytes enlarge and the joint space narrows. Motion limitation of the first MTPJ can be detected with open kinetic chain motion.

The pathomechanical mechanisms have not been fully elucidated with this condition. It seems that coupled with the pronation moment and good hallux alignment there is excessive preload on the medial column and premature engagement of the plantar fascia during early propulsion. If the proximal phalangeal dorsal rim cannot clear the metatarsal head as the windlass engages, then the metatarsal head impinges

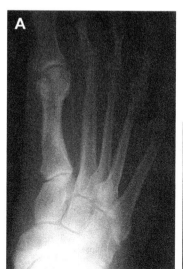
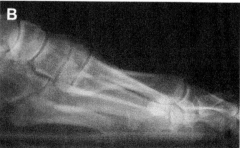

Fig. 11. (*A*) Postoperative radiographs of metatarsal base osteotomy shows first metatarsal shortening and second metatarsal thickening. (*B*) Demonstrates example of iatrogenic distal FR elevation.

on the dorsal rim of the phalanx and bind the joint. This causes increased load on the proximal phalanx.

THE FIRST RAY AND FOOT PRONATION

The FR is the medial stabilizer of the foot; through retrograde forces, it balances and supports the sustenaculum tali that is being eccentrically loaded by the talus. In the normal foot, the function of the FR in propulsion is able to resupinate the foot. Kirby[79,80] described projecting the subtalar joint axis anteriorly to the forefoot and noted its extension between the first and second metatarsals. He described ground reactive loads through the first metatarsal capable of generating a supinatory moment of the rearfoot whereas loads applied to any of the lesser metatarsals collectively generate a pronatory moment (**Fig. 12**).[81] In mild pronation, there can be increased ground reactive pressure on the FR. The windlass function can be compromised because in order to achieve the windlass effect the first metatarsal must plantarflex (arch elevation). If the tension generated on the plantar aponeurosis cannot overcome the pronation moment placed on the foot, then the reverse windlass takes over and excessive loads rise on the hallux and the foot is prevented from resupinating. This process can lead to progressive breakdown of the medial column.

In a pathologically pronated foot, the rearfoot everts and the forefoot abducts on the rearfoot. The subtalar joint axis in this setting projects medial to the entire forefoot; thus, load on any of the metatarsal heads generates a pronation moment on the rearfoot.[81] In a study evaluating the windlass in pronated feet, with medially deviated subtalar joint axis, the windlass effect could not be established.[82] Pronatory moments on the forefoot overload the medial column and gradually break down the plantar ligaments and cause segmental malalignment in the sagittal and transverse planes. Equinus can be destructive to normal foot alignment and FR mechanics, forcing the foot to

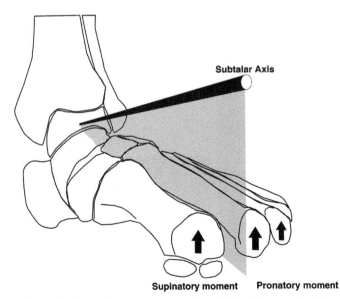

Fig. 12. Illustration of subtalar joint axis in normal position that projects between first and second rays of the forefoot. The first metatarsal is positioned to impart a supinatory moment on the rearfoot, whereas the lesser metatarsal a pronatory moment. A medially deviated subtalar axis would cause all of the metatarsals to impart a pronatory moment.

compensate from body weight, overloading the forefoot and forcing the foot into a pronated position that provides greater dorsiflexion in the midfoot and allows the heel to become plantigrade.

It has been shown that fusion of the first metatarsocuneiform joint has a stabilizing effect to the medial arch.[83,84] When evaluating lateral radiographs, comparing pre- and postoperative images, a reversal of pronation is observed.[83]

SUMMARY

During gait there is more sagittal plane motion in the medial column than in the ankle joint.[30] Normal function of the forefoot in gait relies on, among other factors, load sharing between the metatarsal segments. Balance between the forefoot and rearfoot during gait is created by the FR providing a supination moment and the lesser metatarsals creating a pronation moment relative to the subtalar joint axis. In propulsion, the windlass mechanism stabilizes the FR and induces resupination of the foot. Mechanical insufficiency of the FR should be considered a continuum with variable clinical symptoms and signs appearing as the FR insufficiency worsens. This can be in the form of a short or elevated FR or dorsal hypermobility that occurs dynamically when the first metatarsal segment is not capable of bearing load simultaneously with the second metatarsal. Causes are multifactorial and include ligament deficiencies, windlass delay, and segmental overload. Clinical signs and symptoms of FR pathology should be evaluated collectively, because reliability on one factor or measurement can be misleading as a result of natural variability of the anatomy.

REFERENCES

1. Blackburn MG, Tosh PA, McLeish RD, et al. An investigation of the centres of pressure under the foot while walking. J Bone Joint Surg Br 1975;57:98–103.
2. Hicks JH. Mechanics of the foot 1. The joints. J Anat 1953;87:345–57.
3. Root ML, Orien WP, Weed JH. Motion of the joints of the foot: the first ray. Los Angeles (CA): Clinical Biomechanics Corporation; 1977.
4. Duchenne GB. Physiology of motion. Philadelphia: J.B. Lippincott Co; 1949. (Kaplan EB, Trans. and editor; original work [Physiologie des mouvements] published 1867). p. 612.
5. Lapidus PW. The operative correction of metatarsus varus primus in hallux valgus. Surg Gynecol Obstet 1934;58:183–91.
6. Morton DJ. Metatarsus atavicus: the identification of a distinctive type of foot disorder. J Bone Joint Surg Am 1927;9:531–44.
7. Morton DJ. Hypermobility of the first metatarsal bone. J Bone Joint Surg Am 1928; 10:187–96.
8. Morton DJ. The human foot: its evolution, physiology and functional disorders. Morningside Heights, New York: Columbia University Press; 1935.
9. Morton DJ, Fuller DD. Human locomotion and body form: a study of gravity and man. 1st edition. Baltimore: Williams & Wilkins Company; 1952.
10. Khaw FM, Mak P, Johnson GR, et al. Distal ligamentous restraints of the first metatarsal. An in vitro biomechanical study. Clin Biomech (Bristol, Avon) 2005;20: 653–8.
11. Sarrafian SK. Anatomy of the foot and ankle. 1st edition. Philadelphia: J.B. Lippincott Company; 1983.
12. Sarrafian SK. Functional characteristics of the foot and plantar aponeurosis under tibiotalar loading. Foot Ankle 1987;8:4–18.

13. Hicks JH. The mechanics of the foot: II. The plantar aponeurosis and the arch. J Anat 1954;88:25–30.

14. Thordarson DB, Schmotzer H, Chon J, et al. Dynamic support of the human longitudinal arch. A biomechanical evaluation. Clin Orthop 1995;316:165–72.

15. Johnson CH, Christensen JC. Biomechanics of the first ray. Part I. The effects of peroneus longus function: a three-dimensional kinematic study on a cadaver model. J Foot Ankle Surg 1999;38:313–21.

16. Perez HR, Reber LK, Christensen JC. The effect of frontal plane position on first ray motion: forefoot locking mechanism. Foot Ankle Int 2008;29:72–6.

17. Sharkey NA, Ferris L, Smith TS, et al. Strain and loading of the second metatarsal during heel-lift. J Bone Joint Surg Am 1995;77:1050–7.

18. Stokes IA, Hutton WC, Stott JR. Forces acting on the metatarsals during normal walking. J Anat 1979;129:579–90.

19. Mann R, Inman VT. Phasic activity of intrinsic muscles of the foot. J Bone Joint Surg Am 1964;46:469–81.

20. Carlson RE, Fleming LL, Hutton WC. The biomechanical relationship between the tendoachilles, plantar fascia and metatarsophalangeal joint dorsiflexion angle. Foot Ankle Int 2000;21:18–25.

21. Erdemir A, Hamel AJ, Fauth AR, et al. Dynamic loading of the plantar aponeurosis in walking. J Bone Joint Surg Am 2004;86-A:546–52.

22. Saam JA, Christensen JC, Crawford ME. The effect of gasto-soleal equinus on tension in the plantar fascia—a cadaveric investigation. Presented at the 63rd Annual Meeting of the American College of Foot & Ankle Surgeons. New Orleans, LA, 2005.

23. Huang CK, Kitaoka HB, An KN, et al. Biomechanical evaluation of longitudinal arch stability. Foot Ankle Clin 1993;14:353–7.

24. Rush SM, Christensen JC, Johnson CH. Biomechanics of the first ray. Part II: metatarsus primus varus as a cause of hypermobility. A three-dimensional kinematic analysis in a cadaver model. J Foot Ankle Surg 2000;39:68–77.

25. Weijers RE, Walenkamp GH, van Mameren H, et al. The relationship of the position of the metatarsal heads and peak plantar pressure. Foot Ankle Int 2003;24: 349–53.

26. Cheng HY, Lin CL, Chou SW, et al. Nonlinear finite element analysis of the plantar fascia due to the windlass mechanism. Foot Ankle Int 2008;29:845–51.

27. Daly PJ, Kitaoka HB, Chao EYS. Plantar fasciotomy for intractable plantar fasciitis: clinical results and biomechanical evaluation. Foot Ankle 1992;13:188–95.

28. Erdemir A, Piazza SJ. Changes in foot loading following plantar fasciotomy: a computer modeling study. J Biomech Eng 2004;126:237–43.

29. Nester C, Jones RK, Liu A, et al. Foot kinematics during walking measured using bone and surface mounted markers. J Biomech 2007;40:3412–23.

30. Lundgren P, Nester C, Liu A, et al. Invasive in vivo measurement of rear-, mid- and forefoot motion during walking. Gait Posture 2008;28:93–100.

31. Inman VT, Ralston HJ, Todd F. Human walking. Baltimore (MD): Williams and Wilkins; 1981.

32. Barnett CH. The phases of human gait. Lancet 1956;2:617–21.

33. Collis WJMP, Jayson MIV. Measurement of pedal pressures. Ann Rheum Dis 1972;31:215–7.

34. Elftman H. A cinematic study of the distribution of pressure in the human foot. Anat Rec 1934;59:481–91.

35. Grieve DW, Rashdi T. Pressures under normal feet in standing and walking as measured by foil pedobarography. Ann Rheum Dis 1984;43:816–8.

36. Hutton WC, Dhanendran M. A study of the distribution of load under the normal foot during walking. Int Orthop 1979;3:153–7.
37. Stott JR, Hutton WC, Stokes IA. Forces under the foot. J Bone Joint Surg Br 1973; 55:335–44.
38. Myerson MS, Badekas A. Hypermobility of the first ray. Foot Ankle Clin 2000;5: 469–84.
39. Sangeorzan BJ, Hansen ST Jr. Modified Lapidus procedure for hallux valgus. Foot Ankle 1989;9:262–6.
40. Wukich DK, Donley BG, Sferra JJ. Hypermobility of the first tarsometatarsal joint. Foot Ankle Clin 2005;10:157–66.
41. Davitt JS, Kadel N, Sangeorzan BJ, et al. An association between functional second metatarsal length and midfoot arthrosis. J Bone Joint Surg Am 2005; 87:795–800.
42. Faber FW, Kleinrensink GJ, Mulder PG, et al. Mobility of the first tarsometatarsal joint in hallux valgus patients: a radiographic analysis. Foot Ankle Int 2001;22: 965–9.
43. Grebing BR, Coughlin MJ. Evaluation of Morton's theory of second metatarsal hypertrophy. J Bone Joint Surg Am 2004;86:1375–86.
44. Prieskorn DW, Mann RA, Fritz G. Radiographic assessment of the second metatarsal: measure of first ray hypermobility. Foot Ankle Int 1996;17:331–3.
45. Morton DJ. Mechanism of the normal foot and of flat foot. Part I. J Bone Joint Surg 1924;6:368–86.
46. Morton DJ. Mechanism of the normal foot and of flat foot. Part II. J Bone Joint Surg 1924;6:386–406.
47. Bednarz PA, Manoli A 2nd. Modified lapidus procedure for the treatment of hypermobile hallux valgus. Foot Ankle Int 2000;21:816–21.
48. Coughlin MJ, Jones CP. Hallux valgus and first ray mobility. A prospective study. J Bone Joint Surg Am 2007;89:1887–98.
49. Coughlin MJ, Jones CP, Viladot R, et al. Hallux valgus and first ray mobility: a cadaveric study. Foot Ankle Int 2004;25:537–44.
50. Faber FW, Kleinrensink GJ, Verhoog MW, et al. Mobility of the first tarsometatarsal joint in relation to hallux valgus deformity: anatomical and biomechanical aspects. Foot Ankle Int 1999;20:651–6.
51. Fritz GR, Prieskorn D. First metatarsocuneiform motion: a radiographic and statistical analysis. Foot Ankle Int 1995;16:117–23.
52. Glasoe WM, Allen MK, Ludewig PM. Comparison of first ray dorsal mobility among different forefoot alignments. J Orthop Sports Phys Ther 2000;30: 612–20 [discussion: 21–3].
53. Glasoe WM, Allen MK, Saltzman CL. First ray dorsal mobility in relation to hallux valgus deformity and first intermetatarsal angle. Foot Ankle Int 2001;22:98–101.
54. Glasoe WM, Allen MK, Saltzman CL, et al. Comparison of two methods used to assess first-ray mobility. Foot Ankle Int 2002;23:248–52.
55. Glasoe WM, Grebing BR, Beck S, et al. A comparison of device measures of dorsal first ray mobility. Foot Ankle Int 2005;26:957–61.
56. Glasoe WM, Yack HJ, Saltzman CL. Measuring first ray mobility with a new device. Arch Phys Med Rehabil 1999;80:122–4.
57. Klaue K, Hansen ST, Masquelet AC. Clinical, quantitative assessment of first tarsometatarsal mobility in the sagittal plane and its relation to hallux valgus deformity. Foot Ankle Int 1994;15:9–13.
58. Lee KT, Young K. Measurement of first-ray mobility in normal vs. hallux valgus patients. Foot Ankle Int 2001;22:960–4.

59. Roling BA, Christensen JC, Johnson CH. Biomechanics of the first ray. Part IV: the effect of selected medial column arthrodeses. A three-dimensional kinematic analysis in a cadaver model. J Foot Ankle Surg 2002;41:278–85.

60. Wanivenhaus A, Pretterklieber M. First tarsometatarsal joint: anatomical biomechanical study. Foot Ankle Clin 1989;9:153–7.

61. Wright DG, Rennels DC. A study of the elastic properties of plantar fascia. J Bone Joint Surg 1964;3:482–92.

62. Allen MK, Cuddeford TJ, Glasoe WM, et al. Relationship between static mobility of the first ray and first ray, midfoot, and hindfoot motion during gait. Foot Ankle Int 2004;25:391–6.

63. Christensen JC. Lapidus arthrodesis and firstray hypermobility. Presented at the AO/ASIF COmprehensive Foot & Ankle Course. Colorado Springs, CO, November, 1996.

64. Johnson CH, Christensen JC. Lapidus arthrodesis. Presented at the Annual Meeting of the American Podiatric Medical Association. Seattle, WA, August 17, 2002 [video].

65. Lapidus PW. A quarter of a century of experience with the operative correction of the metatarsus varus in hallux valgus. Bull Hosp Jt Dis Orthop Inst 1956;17:404–21.

66. Lapidus PW. The authors bunion operation from 1931 to 1959. Clin Orthop 1960;16:119–35.

67. Palladino SJ. Preoperative evaluation of the bunion patient: etiology, biomechanics, clinical and radiographic assessment. In: Gerbert J, editor. Textbook of bunion surgery. 2nd edition. Mount Kisco (NY): Futura Publishing Company; 1991. p. 1–79.

68. Weber AK, Hatch DJ, Jensen JL. Use of the first ray splay test to assess transverse plane instability before metatarsocuneiform fusion. J Foot Ankle Surg 2006;45:278–82.

69. Johnson KA, Kile TA. Hallux valgus due to cuneiform-metatarsal instability. J South Ortop Assoc 1994;3:273–82.

70. Romash MM, Fugate D, Yanklowit B. Passive motion of the first metatarsal cuneiform joint: preoperative assessment. Foot Ankle Clin 1990;10:293–8.

71. Shereff MJ, Baumhauer JF. Hallux rigidus and osteoarthrosis of the first metatarsophalangeal joint. J Bone Joint Surg Am 1998;80:898–908.

72. Stokes IA, Hutton WC, Evans MJ. The effects of hallux valgus and Keller's operation on the load-bearing function of the foot during walking. Acta Orthop Belg 1975;41:695–704.

73. Danon G, Pokrassa M. An unusual complication of the Keller bunionectomy: spontaneous stress fractures of all lesser metatarsals. J Foot Surg 1989;28:335–9.

74. Zechman JS. Stress fracture of the second metatarsal after Keller bunionectomy. J Foot Surg 1984;23:63–5.

75. Toth K, Huszanyik I, Kellermann P, et al. The effect of first ray shortening in the development of metatarsalgia in the second through fourth rays after metatarsal osteotomy. Foot Ankle Int 2007;28:61–3.

76. Brodsky JW, Beischer AD, Robinson AH, et al. Surgery for hallux valgus with proximal crescentic osteotomy causes variable postoperative pressure patterns. Clin Orthop Relat Res 2006;443:280–6.

77. Roukis TS, Jacobs PM, Dawson DM, et al. A prospective comparison of clinical, radiographic, and intra-operative features of hallux rigidus: short-term follow-up and analysis. J Foot Ankle Surg 2002;41:158–65.

78. Roukis TS, Jacobs PM, Dawson DM, et al. A prospective comparison of clinical, radiographic, and intra-operative features of hallux rigidus. J Foot Ankle Surg 2002;41:76–95.
79. Kirby KA. Methods for determination of positional variations in the subtalar joint axis. J Am Podiatr Med Assoc 1987;77:228–34.
80. Kirby KA. Rotational equilibrium across the subtalar joint axis. J Am Podiatr Med Assoc 1989;79:1–14.
81. Kirby KA. Subtalar joint axis location and rotational equilibrium theory of foot function. J Am Podiatr Med Assoc 2001;91:465–87.
82. Aquino A, Payne C. Function of the windlass mechanism in excessively pronated feet. J Am Podiatr Med Assoc 2001;91:245–50.
83. Avino A, Patel S, Hamilton GA, et al. The effect of the lapidus arthrodesis on medial longitudinal arch: a radiographic review. J Foot Ankle Surg 2008;47: 510–4.
84. Bierman RA, Christensen JC, Johnson CH. Biomechanics of the first ray. Part III. Consequences of Lapidus arthrodesis on peroneus longus function: a three-dimensional kinematic analysis in a cadaver model. J Foot Ankle Surg 2001;40: 125–31.

Naviculocuneiform Arthrodesis for Treatment of Medial Column Instability Associated with Lateral Peritalar Subluxation

Shannon M. Rush, DPM, FACFAS[a],*, Thomas Jordan, DPM[b]

KEYWORDS

- Naviculocuneiform arthrodesis • Lateral peritalar subluxation
- First ray • Hypermobility

Medial column instability is a common and often complex condition that manifests as many associated clinical disorders. Progressive instability of the medial column usually is the result of equinus contracture, which leads to pathologic midfoot compensation. Morton described medial column insufficiency leading to abnormal pronation, medial deviation of the talus with a shift in the weight-bearing axis of the foot, and increased forces on the posterior tibial tendon.[1] Morton's qualitative descriptions were the earliest and to date the most accurate clinical description of medial column pathomechanics (**Fig. 1**). Medial column instability and progressive collapse of the medial longitudinal arch, dorsiflexion and abduction of the forefoot on the hindfoot, and progressive valgus deformity in the subtalar joint are best described as dorsolateral peritalar subluxation (**Fig. 2**).[2] Various degrees of sagittal, frontal, and transverse plane deformity exist creating different clinical and radiographic manifestations of the collapsed arch. The etiology is believed to be a combination of factors, including equinus contracture, congenital configuration of the anatomic osseous structure, and insufficiency of the dynamic (posterior tibial tendon and peroneus longus) and static soft tissue stabilizers (plantar ligaments) of the arch.[3–16] Other popular descriptors of this condition are adult acquired flatfoot or posterior tibial tendon dysfunction.[9,12] The problem with these descriptions is that not all symptomatic flatfeet have posterior tibial tendon pathology. Often, the severe instability in the arch and hindfoot valgus result in significant arch fatigue, functional foot pain, sinus tarsi

[a] Department of Orthopedics and Podiatric Surgery, The Palo Alto Medical Foundation, Camino Division, 701 El Camino Real, Mountain View, CA 94040, USA
[b] San Francisco Bay Area Foot and Ankle Residency Program, San Francisco, CA, USA
* Corresponding author.
E-mail address: rushdoc@gmail.com (S.M. Rush).

Clin Podiatr Med Surg 26 (2009) 373–384
doi:10.1016/j.cpm.2009.03.008
0891-8422/09/$ – see front matter © 2009 Elsevier Inc. All rights reserved.

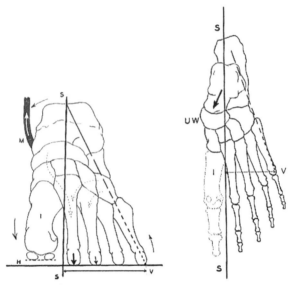

Fig. 1. Medial column insufficiency, as described by Morton, leads to lateral shift of weight-bearing axis of the foot, abnormal pronatory forces, medial deviation of the talus, and additional mechanical load on the posterior tibial tendon (*From* Morton DJ. The human foot: its evolution, physiology and functional disorders. New York: Columbia University Press; 1935; with permission).

pain, and subfibular impingement. These symptoms often bring patients to seek help as often as for posterior tibial tendon pathology.

The structural support of the medial column plays a vital role in maintaining a stable lever between the fulcrum of the forefoot and the primary input effort of the Achilles

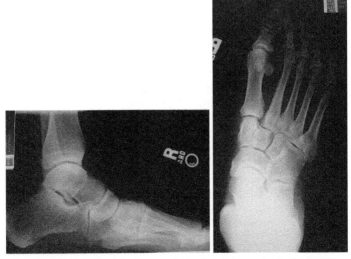

Fig. 2. Medial column fault. This results from pathologic compensation in the medial column from ankle equines. As instability in the medial column progresses, the support of the talar head by virtue of the navicular articulation is compromised. Lateral midtarsal subluxation results. Note the talar head coverage, talocalcaneal angle, and talometatarsal axis on the anteroposterior film.

tendon. This class II lever creates a bending moment through the midfoot. Ideally, in any lever system there should be no instability in the lever arm. The ability to withstand this bending moment is established by the osseous architechture of the midfoot, ligamentous structures (in particular the plantar ligaments), dynamic support via the posterior tibial tendon, and to a lessor degree the peroneus longus. Stokes and colleagues[17] demonstrated that the medial column is subject to an upward shear force and bending moment in the dorsiflexion direction throughout forefoot contact with the ground and these calculated forces were found highest for the first metatarsal. Disruption of this critical equilibrium leads to progressive arch collapse and mechanical insufficiency in the medial column. Johnson and Christensen[18] further demonstrated the arch-lowering effect the Achilles tendon has on the medial column of the foot. The terms, *lateral subluxation* and *dorsolateral peritalar subluxation*, are used to describe the acquired flatfoot deformity as the hindfoot rotates about the talus.[2] This functional description of the pathologic subluxation of the foot relative to the talus, which is fixed in the ankle mortise, is an accurate and reliable way to characterize this condition. Degenerative arthritis and adaptive joint stiffness are predictable consequences of longstanding deformity but are only variations of the same pathologic process. Greisberg and colleagues[19] showed that medial column fusion realigns hindfoot radiographic correction of peritalar subluxation in the sagittal and transverse planes (**Fig. 3**).

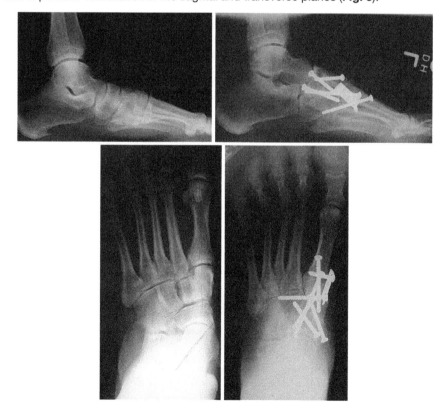

Fig. 3. Lateral peritalar subluxation. Medial column insufficiency with uncovering of talar head and subtalar joint valgus. Note the position of the lateral process of the talus pre- and postoperatively. Stabilizing the pathologic medial column insufficiency and equines contracture corrects any pathologic hindfoot compensation. The talometatarsal axis and talar head coverage has been restored.

The clinical manifestations usually include the development of functional foot pain, poor walking and standing endurance, and slowly progressive flattening of the arch. As medial column instability progresses, hindfoot subluxation ensues leading to lateral peritalar subluxation. In addition, with the development of hindfoot pathomechanics, increased functional loads are placed on the posterior tibial tendon, which often leads to dysfunction and secondary tendon pathology. The exact chronology of posterior tibial tendon pathology is not well documented. The authors believe it is rare to see degenerative posterior tibial tendon pathology without some degree of medial column instability and equinus contracture.

In a cadaveric study, Roling and colleagues[20] demonstrated that the naviculocuneiform joint (NCJ) joint contributes an average of 50% total first ray sagittal plane motion whereas the metatarsocuneiform joint (MCJ) and talonavicular joint (TNJ) contribute 41% and 9%, respectively. Their findings explain in part the various clinical and radiographic manifestations of the same condition foot and ankle surgeons encounter with medial column instability. Johnson and Christensen demonstrated the effects the peroneus longus had on the medial column. They showed the peroneus longus created an eversion locking mechanism which stabilizes the medial column.[21] In addition, they demonstrated the dampening effect the Achilles tendon had on peroneus longus function. This finding supports the philosophy that the Achilles tendon can have a degenerative effect on the dynamic supporting structures on the medial column, namely the peroneus longus and posterior tibial tendon.

Radiographically, lateral peritalar subluxation can be evaluated by multiple criteria. The talometatarsal axis on the anteroposterior and lateral projections demonstrates the degree of dorsolateral drift of the forefoot. Talonavicular coverage in addition to the talocancaneal angle gives an indication of hindfoot instability at the level of the midtarsal joint. Hindfoot deformity can be assessed with long leg calcaneal axial and hindfoot alignment views. These views allow assessment of valgus angulation and lateral subluxation in the subtalar joint, respectively (**Fig. 4**). Chi and colleagues[8]

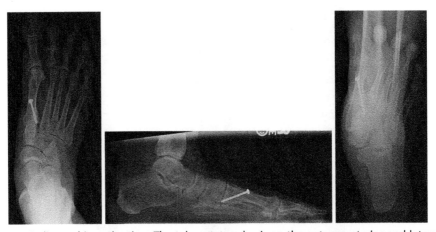

Fig. 4. Radiogrpahic evaluation. The talometatarsal axis on the anteroposterior and lateral projections demonstrates the degree of dorsolateral drift of the forefoot. Talonavicular coverage in addition to the talocancaneal angle gives an indication of hindfoot instability at the level of the midtarsal joint. Hindfoot deformity can be assessed with long leg calcaneal axial or hindfoot alignment views. These views allow assessment of valgus angulation and lateral subluxation in the subtalar joint, respectively.

reported a decrease lateral talometatarsal angle and talonavicular coverage angle of 20° and 10°, respectively, in 5 feet that received fusions of the NCJ or first MCJ. Greisberg and colleagues[19] reported improvements in the lateral talometatarsal angle and talonavicular coverage of 16° and 14°, respectively, in 13 feet that received fusions of the NCJ and first MCJ and 3 feet that received a fusion of the first MCJ. These studies support the reasoning that by stabilizing the primary biomechanical dysfunction of the medial column, the lateral peritalar subluxation deformity can be improved.

The first tarsomatatarsal joint often is included in the medial column stabilization. The indications for additional tarsometatarsal arthrodesis are first ray deformity with instability (**Fig. 5**). Stabilizing the medial column restores the stable lever arm mechanics of the arch and weight-bearing axis of the foot, as described by Morton,[1] and secondarily restores stability to the midtarsal joint. In the sagittal plane, the improved alignment is evidenced by restoration of the talometatarsal axis and improved talonavicular coverage. Hindfoot foot valgus also is restored with the condition that there is sufficient mobility in the joint to allow correction. The hindfoot alignment must be assessed carefully on the operating table. Intraoperative hindfoot views are helpful to assess the position of the calcaneus relative to the tibial axis. Any residual hindfoot valgus or lateral translation should be addressed with a medializing calcaneal osteotomy.

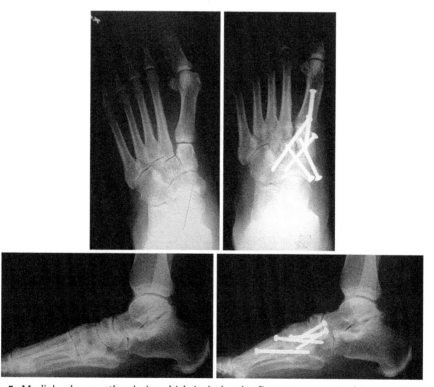

Fig. 5. Medial column arthrodesis, which includes the first tarsometatarsal joint. Note the associated first ray deformity with elevation and subtle plantar gapping at the tarsometatarsal joint. These findings are diagnostic for mechanical instability in the medial column and criteria for inclusion in the arthorodesis. Note the restoration of the talometarsal axis, talar head coverage, and hindfoot position with medial column stabilization.

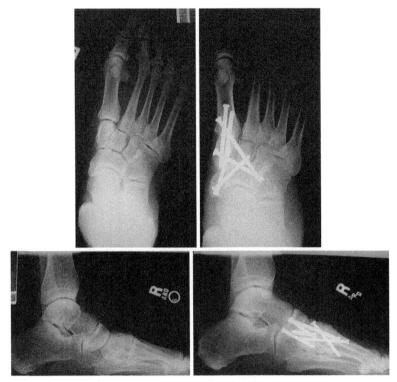

Fig. 5. (*continued*)

Greisberg and colleagues hypothesized that hindfoot valgus has a forefoot origin, which occurs secondary to with TNJ subluxation, explaining that the medial column acts as a post or buttress for the talus. By restoring the medial support, the talar alignment is corrected.[19] Therefore, the hindfoot valgus, which results from the insufficient medial column, can be considered a forefoot-driven hindfoot valgus.

OPERATIVE TECHNIQUE

A gastrocnemius recession or a percutaneous TAL procedure is routinely performed on all patients based on the patient's preoperative Silfverskiold test. If a percutaneous tendoachilles lengthening (TAL) is to be performed, this procedure is done last. The authors believe that a more precise evaluation of the equinus contracture can be appreciated after the deformity has been corrected.

Proper exposure of the NCJ is the most critical aspect of a successful operation. The approach to the medial column is done through the medial utility incision advocated by Hansen[2] (**Fig. 6**). The incision is centered over the medial column of the foot just inferior to the dorsal venous arch medial dorsal cutaneous nerve. The incision can be extended proximal and distal to include additional exposure to the posterior tibial tendon and the first tarsometatarsal joint. Adequate exposure allows a surgeon to visualize all three cuneiform facets (**Fig. 7**). Exposure, débridement, and preparation of all three articular facets play a critical role in for optimal correction. This can easily be accomplished with release of the dorsal and plantar ligaments. The authors prefer a Weinraub retractor to facilitate exposure of the joint for arthrodesis. The articular

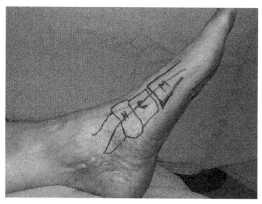

Fig. 6. The approach to the medial column is done through the medial utility incision, advocated by Hansen.[2] The incision is centered over the medial column of the foot just inferior to the dorsal venous arch medial dorsal cutaneous nerve. The incision can be extended proximal and distal to include additional exposure to the posterior tibial tendon or tarsometatarsal joint. This medial exposure facilitates placement of internal fixation.

cartilage and the subchondral bone are removed. Often the navicular facet is dense and sclerotic and the subchondral must be removed to ensure a high rate of arthrodesis. After removal of the subchondral bone, fish scaling is preformed before reduction and fixation. Fish scaling of the arthrodesis site serves two important purposes. It increases the surface area of the arthrodesis site and acts as a small autogenous bone graft, which creates a local, shear-strain bone graft technique (**Fig. 8**).[18] Using a saw to remove the articular surfaces of the NCJ requires a significant amount of resection to achieve removal of all three facets. Excessive removal of bone from either side of the arthrodesis site can make placement and stability of internal fixation difficult.

Reduction of the arthrodesis site should be accomplished on a preliminary basis and alignment verified visually and with intraoperative imaging. Reduction can be facilitated by a large tenaculum (**Fig. 9**). The large tenaculum affords excellent

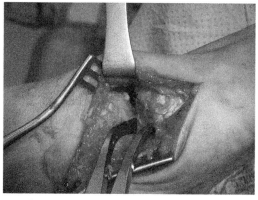

Fig. 7. The NCJ is exposed with release of the dorsal and plantar ligaments. A distractor is used for exposure. The lateral cuneiform should be visualized ensuring a complete debridement of all the articular surfaces.

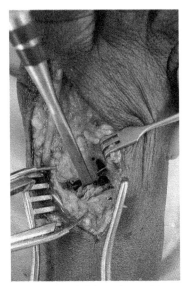

Fig. 8. Removal of subchondral bone and fish scaling. This acts as a local bone graft and increases the surface area of the arthrodesis. The Weinraub retractor helps with exposure of the joint.

compression across the arthrodesis site. One end of the clamp is placed on the navicular tuberosity and the other end on the dorsal first cuneiform. As the clamp is reduced the cuneiform articulations are translated medial and plantar relative to the navicular. A slight forefoot valgus is the ideal position to achieve. A gap at the dorsal aspect of the NCJ often is seen after reduction, which is not uncommon in longstanding cases resulting from adapted or degenerative changes in the midfoot (**Fig. 10**). Backfilling of the dorsal void with bone graft can remedy this small amount of gapping.

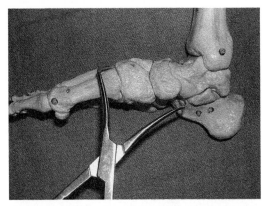

Fig. 9. Reduction can be facilitated by a large tenaculum. The large tenaculum affords excellent compression across the arthrodesis site. One end of the clamp is placed on the navicular tuberosity and the other end on the dorsal first cuneiform. As the clamp is reduced, the cuneiform articulations are translated medial and plantar relative to the navicular. A slight forefoot valgus is the ideal position to achieve.

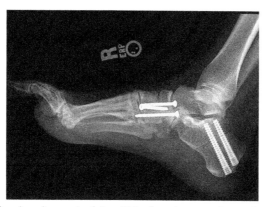

Fig. 10. A gap at the dorsal aspect of the NCJ often is seen after reduction, which is not uncommon in longstanding cases because of adapted or degenerative changes in the mid-foot. There is no clinical consequence to this finding as long as the joint is well reduced and stable internal fixation is achieved. Generally the plantar two thirds of the joint are all that is needed for a successful arthrodesis.

Fixation can be accomplished in several ways but there are two techniques the authors believe give reliable results. Cortical lag screw fixation is a reliable technique that affords excellent stability at the arthrodesis site and achieves reliable results. The authors prefer stacked screws from plantar to dorsal (see **Figs. 3** and **5**) The preference is for a 4.0 mm cortical screw, which has a larger core diameter, or a 3.5 mm cortical screw. With the reduction clamp in place, the first screw is placed from the navicular tuberosity just superior to the insertion of the posterior tibial tendon into the plantar third medial cuneiform. A second screw is placed from the dorsomedial navicular into the second cuneiform. A third screw is placed through a small incision made in the tibialis anterior tendon just proximal to the tarsometatarsal joint. The third screw is aimed at the lateral navicular body. Intraopertive imaging can verify the reduction and placement of fixation. Evaluation of fixation on the anteroposterior and lateral views is critical in assessing screw placement into the navicular as the cup-shaped architecture of the TNJ can give the appearance that the screws violate the TNJ on the anteriposterior view. Alternatively, plate fixation is stable and reliable fixation technique. A medially placed cervical H-plate works well. Various forms of this plate are available with some designed with locking plate technology. Axial compression is not obtained as easily from a plate so reduction and compression with the reduction clamp are critical when plating this arthrodesis. The proximal end of the plate should be positioned 1-cm proximal to the NCJ and not on the navicular tuberosity (**Fig. 11**). This plate positioning should ensure the perpendicular screws placed through the plate do not violate the TNJ and gain optimal purchase in the navicular body. Ideally the screws in the proximal end of the plate are just distal to the TNJ and span the medial to lateral width of the navicular body. Distal fixation is secured into the cuneiforms. Placing screws across the intercuneiform joints is acceptable and allows for better distal fixation.

Radiographic correction after NCJ arthrodesis can be accomplished in all three planes. The most dramatic correction is seen in the talometatarsal axis on the anteroposterior and lateral views. Transverse plane correction with improved talar head coverage is predictable and traditionally believed possible only with lateral column

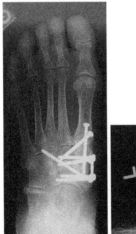
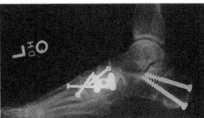

Fig. 11. Medial plate fixation. The proximal end of the plate should be positioned 1-cm proximal to the NCJ and not on the navicular tuberosity. This plate positioning should ensure that the perpendicular screws placed through the plate do not violate the TNJ and gain optimal purchase in the navicular body. Ideally, the screws in the proximal end of the plate are just distal to the TNJ and span the medial to lateral width of the navicular body. Distal fixation is secured into the cuneiforms. Placing screws across the intercuneiform joints is acceptable and allows for better distal fixation.

lengthening. Sagittal plane correction of the medial column fault is evident as is a restoration of midtarsal joint alignment and calcaneal inclination.

Postoperatively the foot and ankle are immobilized in a short leg cast for 6 weeks with touch-down weight bearing. Radiographs are taken at 6 weeks and patients are progressed to full weight bearing and therapy at that time. Rates of successful arthrodesis using stable internal fixation and standard arthrodesis principles are not widely published. The author's unpublished data (Rush SM, DPM, unpublished data, 2009) using this technique show a 3.9% nonunion rate (2/51) using lag screws or medial H-plate internal fixation. One nonunion occurring in a patient who had diabetes and peripheral neuropathy initially was fixed with cortical lag screw technique. Successful revision and union were achieved with distal tibial bone grafting and medial plate fixation. The second nonunion occurred in a patient who had vitamin D deficiency. Initial fixation was achieved with cortical lag screws. Successful revision was accomplished with medial plate fixation, tibial bone grafting, and correction of metabolic deficiency.

SUMMARY

Medial column instability is a common disorder that leads to predictable hindfoot subluxation and posterior tibial tendon dysfunction. Recognizing the medial column as the primary cause of the hindfoot deformity should direct foot and ankle surgeons to choose the best surgical procedure. Addressing soft tissue contracture, such as gastrocnemius equinus, soft tissue adaptation, and motor weakness, restores durability and weight-bearing stability to the arch and hindfoot. Careful attention must be paid to the clinical and radiographic findings seen with this condition as the findings are variable and the decision-making process is critical to the eventual surgical outcome.

REFERENCES

1. Morton DJ, editor. The human foot: its evolution, physiology and functional disorders. New York: Columbia University Press; 1935.
2. Hansen ST Jr. Functional reconstruction of the foot and ankle. Philadelphia: Lippincott Williams and Wilkins; 2000.
3. Hirose CB, Johnsos JE. Plantarflexion opening wedge medial cuneiform osteotomy for correction of fixed forefoot varus associated with flatfoot deformity. Foot Ankle Int 2004;25:568–74.
4. Mann RA, Thompson FM. Rupture of the posterior tibial tendon causing flatfoot. J Bone Joint Surg Am 1985;67:556–61.
5. Hiller L, Pinney SJ. Surgical treatment of acquired flatfoot deformity: what is the state of practice among academic foot and ankle surgeons in 2002? Foot Ankle Int 2003;24:701–5.
6. Pomeroy GC, Pike RH, Beals TC, et al. Acquired flatfoot in adults due to dysfunction of the posterior tibial tendon. J Bone Joint Surg Am 1999;81:1173–82.
7. Ford LA, Hamilton GA. Naviculocuneiform arthrodesis. Clin Podiatr Med Surg 2004;21:141–56.
8. Chi TD, Toolan BC, Sangeorzan BJ, et al. The lateral column lengthening and medial column stabilization procedures. Clin Orthop 1999;365:81–90.
9. Pinney SJ, Lin SS. Current concept review: acquired adult flatfoot deformity. Foot Ankle Int 2006;27:66–74.
10. Greisberg J, Hansen ST, Sangeorzan B. Deformity and degeneration in the hindfoot and midfoot joints of the adult acquired flatfoot. Foot Ankle Int 2003;24:530–4.
11. DiGiovanni CW, Langer P. The role of isolated gastrocnemius and combined Achilles contractures in the flatfoot. Foot Ankle Clin 2007;12:363–79.
12. Myerson MS. Adult acquired flatfoot deformity. J Bone Joint Surg Am 1996;78:780–92.
13. Digiovanni CW, Kuo R, Tejwani N, et al. Isolated gastrocnemius tightness. J Bone Joint Surg Am 2002;84:962–70.
14. Gazdag AR, Carcchiolo A. Rupture of the posterior tibial tendon. Evaluation of injury of the spring ligament and clinical assessment of tendon transfer and ligament repair. J Bone Joint Surg Am 1997;79:675–81.
15. Myerson MS, Badekas A, Schon LC. Treatment of stage II posterior tibial tendon deficiency with flexor digitorum longus tendon transfer and calcaneal osteotomy. Foot Ankle Int 2004;25:445–50.
16. Thordarson DB, Hedman T, Lundquist D, et al. Effect of calcaneal osteotomy and plantar fasciotomy on arch configuration in a flatfoot model. Foot Ankle Int 1998;19:374–8.
17. Stokes IA, Hutton WC, Scott JR. Forces acting on the metatarsals during normal walking. J Anat 1979;129(3):579–90.
18. Johnson CH, Christensen JC. Biomechanics of the first ray part V: the effect of equinus deformity. A 3-dimensional kinematic study on a cadaver model. J Foot Ankle Surg 2005;44(1):114–20.
19. Greisberg J, Assal M, Hansen ST, et al. Isolated medial column stabalization improves alignment in adult-acquired flatfoot. Clin Orthop 2005;435:197–202.
20. Roling BA, Christensen JC, Johnson CH. Biomechanics of the first ray part IV: the effect of selected medial column arthrodesis. A three-dimensional kinematic analysis in a cadaver model. J Foot Ankle Surg 2002;41:278–85.

21. Johnson CH, Christensen JC. Biomechanics of the first ray Part I: the effects of peroneus longus function: a three-dimensional kinematic study on a cadaver model. J Foot Ankle Surg 1999;38(5):313–21.

FURTHER READINGS

Aminian A, Sangeorzan BJ. The anatomy of cavus foot deformity. Foot Ankle Clin 2008;13(2):191–8.

Catanzariti AR, Mendicino RW, Lee MS, et al. The modified Lapidus arthrodesis: a retrospective analysis. J Foot Ankle Surg 1999;38:322–32.

Coetzee JC, resig SG, Kuskowski M, et al. The Lapidus procedure as a salvage after failed surgical treatment of hallux valgus: a prospective cohort study. J Bone Joint Surg Am 2003;85A:60–5.

Cotton FJ. Foot statics and surgery. N Engl J Med 1936;214:353–62.

Fayazi AH, Hoan-Vu N, Juliano PJ. Intermediate term follow-up of calcaneal osteotomy and flexor digitorum longus transfer for treatment of posterior tibial tendon dysfunction. Foot Ankle Int 2002;23:1107–11.

Fraser RK, Menelaus MB, Williams PF, et al. The Miller procedure for mobile flat feet. J Bone Joint Surg Br 1995;77-B(3):396–9.

Gould N. Graphing the adult foot and ankle. Foot Ankle 1982;2:213–9.

Hartog BD. Flexor digitorum longus transfer with medial displacement calcaneal osteotomy: biomechanical rationale. Foot Ankle Clin 2001;6(1):67–76.

Hockenbury RT, Sammarco GJ. Medial sliding calcaneal osteotomy with flexor hallucis longus transfer for the treatment of posterior tibial tendon insufficiency. Foot Ankle Clin 2001;6:569–81.

Malerba F, Fabrizio D. Calcaneal osteotomies. Foot Ankle Clin N Am 2005;10:523–4.

Mann R. Flatfoot in adults. In: Ryan JD, editor. Surgery of the foot and ankle. St Louis (MO): Mosby; 1993. p. 757–84.

McInnes BD, Bouche RT. Critical evaluation of the modified Lapidus procedure. J Foot Ankle Surg 2001;40:71–90.

Miller OL. A plastic flat foot operation. J Bone Joint Surg 1927;9A:84–91.

Myerson MS, Corrigan J. Treatment of posterior tibial tendon dysfunction with flexor digitorum longus tendon transfer and calcaneal osteotomy. Orthopedics 1996;19:383–9.

Myerson MS, Badekas A, Schon LC. Treatment of stage II posterior tibial tendon transfer and calcaneal osteotomy. Foot Ankle Int 2004;25:445–51.

Patel S, Ford LA, Etcheverry J, et al. Modifieds Lapidus arthrodesis: rate of nonunion in 227 cases. J Foot Ankle Surg 2004;43:37–42.

Rush SM, Ford LA, Hamilton GA. Morbidity associated with high gastrocnemius recession: retrospective review of 126 cases. J Foot Ankle Surg 2006;45:156–60.

Sangeorzan BJ, Hansen ST Jr. Modified Lapidus procedure for hallux valgus. Foot Ankle Int 1989;9:262–6.

Sangeorzan BJ, Mosca V, Hansen ST. The effect of calcaneal lengthening on the relationships among the hindfoot, midfoot and forefoot. Foot Ankle Int 1993;14:136–41.

Wacker JT, Hennessy MS, Saxby TS. Calcaneal osteotomy and transfer of the tendon of flexor digitorum longus for stage II dysfunction of tibialis posterior: three to five year results. J Bone Joint Surg Br 2002;84:54–8.

The Impact of the First Ray in the Cavovarus Foot

John M. Schuberth, DPM[a],*, Nina Babu-Spencer, DPM[b]

KEYWORDS

- Cavus • First ray • Metatarsal • Tendon transfer
- Jones suspension

The impact of the first ray on the pathogenesis and maintenance of cavovarus deformity is profound. Although mediated by intrinsic and extrinsic muscle imbalances, the propagation of cavovarus foot deformity by the first ray position is unique because of the antigravity phenomenon. The obligate plantar-flexed position of the first ray in the cavovarus foot can be causative and adaptive in almost all cases.

To understand the cascade-like effect of the first ray on the architectural morphology of the cavovarus foot, it is useful to adopt the notion that the foot is essentially supported by three points of contact that include the first and fifth metatarsal heads and the calcaneus (**Fig. 1**). These three points of contact were coined the "static triangle of support" by Cotton[1] more than 70 years ago. For reasons unknown, this concept has not been applied clinically to the cavovarus foot. Yet, when one expands the notion, it serves as the fundamental premise of this intriguing deformity.

If one considers the three points of contact and the superincumbent foot as a flexible tripod, it becomes easier to understand the architectural change over time that typifies the cavovarus foot. Although the cavus foot is most commonly characterized as a rigid unyielding structure, it becomes clear with empiric observation that this is not the case. The apex of the flexible tripod is located at or close to the center of the midtarsal joint, or just lateral to the talonavicular joint.[2–4] As the foot morphology adapts to the progressive plantar flexion of the first ray, the apex becomes more cephalad and lateral and the distance between the first metatarsal head and calcaneus diminishes, proportionate to the degree of plantar deviation of the first ray. As the severity of the deformity increases, however, the distance between the fifth metatarsal and the calcaneus usually remains static in the cavovarus foot but can decrease in the purely cavoid foot. Torsional deformation is fundamental to the concept of the flexible tripod as a model for the cavovarus foot. With progression of the first ray plantar flexion, the

[a] Foot and Ankle Surgery, Department of Orthopedic Surgery, Kaiser Foundation Hospital, 450 6th Avenue, San Francisco, CA 94118, USA
[b] Kaiser San Francisco Bay Area Foot and Ankle Residency Program, Kaiser Foundation Hospital, Oakland, CA, USA
* Corresponding author.
E-mail address: jmfoot@aol.com (J.M. Schuberth).

Clin Podiatr Med Surg 26 (2009) 385–393
doi:10.1016/j.cpm.2009.04.001
0891-8422/09/$ – see front matter © 2009 Elsevier Inc. All rights reserved.

podiatric.theclinics.com

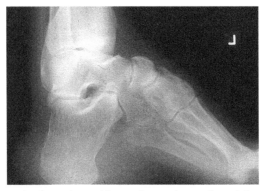

Fig.1. Lateral radiograph of a patient with an advanced cavus foot deformity. Note the three points of contact of the heel and the first and fifth metatarsal heads.

foot undergoes a tridimensional torsion that distorts the normal structural relations and complicates the surgical reversal of the osseous malposition (**Fig. 2**).

The observation that arch height actually increases against the forces of gravity and superincumbent body weight should suggest that this condition is progressive. The progressive nature of the deformity is driven by muscle imbalance that can be obvious, subtle, or even occult. As such, formulation of a surgical plan should incorporate procedures that attempt to mitigate dynamic muscular imbalances. Furthermore, patient expectations should be tempered with respect to the longevity of corrective surgery, particularly if the muscular forces are not completely recognized or neutralized. In particular, in those patients with mild muscular deficiencies or imbalances, the identification of the precise dynamic deformation may not be possible. Furthermore, the neurologic presentation of each patient is individualistic and is not able to be compartmentalized into a recognized disease or syndrome. As such, universal application of finite surgical procedures is not possible.

The definitive position of the first ray has the most impact on the final morphology of the foot and, ultimately, on the function of the extremity after surgical correction. Accordingly, understanding the muscular influences on the first ray is critical to formulation of a surgical plan. There are two primary movers of the first ray, the peroneus longus and tibialis anterior, and one secondary mover, the distal extensions of the posterior tibial tendon. In addition, the first ray is influenced indirectly by the long extensor and flexor of the great toe, the peroneus brevis, and, to a lesser extent,

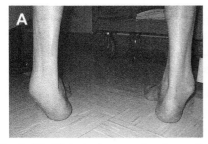
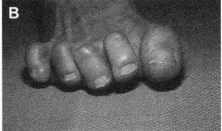

Fig. 2. (*A*) Clinical photograph of a patient who has neuromuscular disease and long-standing cavus. Note the torsion of the entire foot around the talus. (*B*) View of a different patient shows the torsion of the digits with developmental cavus.

the long lesser toe extrinsics and the digital intrinsic muscles. The dynamics and interplay among the various components have been well explained but can be distilled down to the following clinically useful tenet. In the cavus foot, as the first ray migrates plantarly, it causes a commensurate retrograde supinatory coil of the rest of the foot (see **Fig. 2**).[5–10]

Surgical treatment of the cavovarus foot is complex and can often involve more segments than just the obvious deformities of the foot. This discussion focuses on the first ray, recognizing that it is clearly inadequate to treat the cavovarus foot with such an isolationist technique. In fact, one should probably consider the manipulation of the first ray as merely a component, albeit a critical one, of the surgical rehabilitation of the cavovarus foot. Failure to correct any muscle imbalances or suprastructural malalignments diminishes the likelihood of long-term patient satisfaction and a static plantigrade foot.

Another complicating factor in some of these seemingly idiopathic presentations of cavus foot is the difficulty in establishing the true neuromuscular parameters. Intuitively, it would seem that arch height and morphology are determined by genetic predisposition simply as an individual characteristic much like eye color or stature. It would follow that those patients who present with a higher arched foot than normal would maintain that same arch contour throughout life. Empiric clinical observation indicates that this situation is distinctly rare, however. Rather, insidious or fulminant progression is far more common. Yet, the rate of the structural change is difficult to establish, even when the underlying cause of the muscular imbalance can be identified and quantitated. Nevertheless, these observations underscore the fact that most cavovarus feet have an underlying neuromuscular imbalance that universally affects the position of the first ray over time.

Another quandary in the assessment of the cavovarus foot is one of flexibility versus rigidity. Surgeons have long thought that flexible malpositions are the prelude to rigid deformities. This notion may not be entirely operational in the cavovarus presentation, however. Clearly, it is exceedingly rare to examine a child with a rigid cavovarus foot, yet not so uncommon to find an adolescent with a stiff cavus foot. The latter is usually the harbinger of more serious neuromuscular disease, but the point is that the crossover point from flexible to rigid is obtuse and cannot be precisely located on the continuum. The real issue is not determining the threshold; rather, it is deciding if surgical intervention during the fluid phase of deformity is likely to thwart the progression of the deformity or development of rigidity. Until such questions are answered, one can only rely on common sense and empiric surveillance.

To decide whether the first ray deformity is rigid or flexible, there are several important maneuvers to execute. The first clinical determinant is the Coleman block test. This helps to establish the role of the first ray with regard to the varus position of the calcaneus and the flexibility of the hindfoot.[11] If it is determined that the hindfoot varus is clearly forefoot driven, surgery on the first ray is obligate. Yet, the converse is probably not universally true in those situations in which the first ray position has not become fixed. It may still be prudent to perform some balancing type procedures that have an impact on the first ray position, even if the first ray has no direct effect on calcaneal varus. Obvious examples include transfer of the peroneus longus to the peroneus brevis, Jones tenosuspension, hallux interphalangeal fusion, and osteotomy or fusion of the first ray itself.

The second clinical maneuver is to load the foot to simulate weight bearing in the operating room or at the preoperative assessment (**Fig. 3**). This better enables one to determine the flexibility of the first ray deformity. In some patients, the first ray is indeed flexible or reducible while sitting on the examination platform. As the foot is

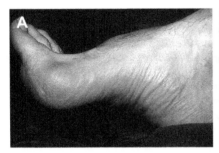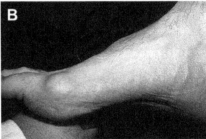

Fig. 3. (*A*) Medial view of a patient with advanced cavus deformity. (*B*) Simulated weight bearing demonstrates considerable reduction of the deformity.

dorsiflexed and everted, the plantar structures become taut and the impact of the peroneus longus on the mobility of the first metatarsal is manifest.[11] Most commonly and importantly, as the foot is placed in this simulated weight-bearing posture, the assumed flexibility is significantly dampened and the plantar flexion deformity seems more profound. This observation should be taken into account when formulating a surgical strategy.

SURGICAL MANIPULATION OF THE FIRST RAY

There are essentially three techniques that can be used to affect the position of the first ray directly. They include dorsiflexion osteotomy, fusion of the first metatarsal cuneiform joint, and tendon transfer. Again, in a large percentage of cases, manipulation of the first ray alone is insufficient to provide a long-lasting, balanced, and plantigrade foot. This capacity for osseous migration over time should be thoroughly explained to the patient before intervention. The uncertainty and incomplete penetration of the underlying neuromuscular condition make any assurances about longevity of correction spurious at best.

Dorsiflexory First Metatarsal Osteotomy

Dorsiflexion osteotomy of the first metatarsal provides the most immediate and obvious correction of the deformity and is relatively easy to perform. The primary objective is to relocate the contact point of the first metatarsal head in a more superior direction. By raising the contact point of the medial column, the foot has the facility to "uncoil" if there is any remaining flexibility, or serves to balance the tripod. Virtually all procedures in the mid- or hindfoot influence the position of the first ray. In particular, any abductory surgical maneuver on the lateral side of the foot exacerbates the plantar-flexed attitude of the first metatarsal. Realignment of the medial osseous structures proximal to the first metatarsal may raise the first metatarsal head superiorly but generally does not affect the angulatory pitch of the bone. In effect, the correction afforded may not be enough to balance the tripod. Regardless, it is prudent to address the first ray as the last procedure of the surgical session. The surgeon can then accurately assess the degree of dorsiflexion necessary to achieve three-point balance.[12,13]

To capitalize on the inherent lever arm of the long first metatarsal, the dorsiflexory osteotomy is performed in the proximal metaphysis. A paramedian incision provides the best exposure and can be developed in isolation or as an extension of the more proximal exposure if available. Subperiosteal dissection is not necessary, and a simple exposure that allows the surgeon to visualize the metaphyseal flare and the insertion of the tibialis anterior is all that is necessary. The orientation of the dorsally based wedge is optional, and good results are obtained when the apex is directly plantar, proximal, or distal (**Fig. 4**). Establishing the apex in the more plastic metaphyseal cortex allows for intraoperative refinement of the ultimate dorsiflexed position of the bone. Successive resections of bone to increase the correction are often necessary, and if the apex was established more distal, the denser plantar cortical bone may fail with repeated manipulations. Conversely, insertion of screw fixation is easiest when delivered from dorsal distal to plantar proximal. Fixation of the completed and opposed osteotomy should provide osseous stability. Most commonly, lag screw fixation oriented perpendicular to the osteotomy is used, but other less rigid fixatives are suitable in view of the obligate non–weight-bearing postoperative course.

Fusion of the First Metatarsal Cuneiform Joint

Fusion of the first metatarsal cuneiform joint also can provide significant change in the position of the first ray.[5] The stability afforded at the fusion site may give the surgeon a false sense of permanency, however. In the face of uncorrected muscle imbalances, migration of the first ray segment can occur over time. Although it is counterintuitive, the overall segment appears to bend as eccentric forces act on the bony segment. This is particularly true when the muscle imbalances are more spastic. Removal of the joint or mobile linkage can perhaps delay the onset of recurrence, but one is cautioned that fusion of the ray does not guarantee that the functional position is not going to change over time. In addition, it has never been established that there is any inherent deformity of the first metatarsal-cuneiform joint that would allow for or cause plantar flexion of the metatarsal through the joint surface in the cavus foot.

The technical aspects of arthrodesis of the first metatarsal cuneiform joint are well described.[14–18] Because this procedure is indicated primarily in such pathologic findings as hallux valgus or first ray hypermobility, the surgical approach most often has been a dorsal one. Although this can still be used in the cavus foot, it is far more difficult to calibrate the amount of bone to be removed to balance the forefoot. An alternative approach is the medial one, which may have already been developed for more proximal procedures of the mid- and hindfoot (**Fig. 5**). From the medial perspective, the surgeon has an easier time quantitating the amount of bone to be removed dorsally. The most common tendency is to remove too much bone, with resultant overcorrection. Yet, this tendency is partially mitigated by a medial exposure. Regardless of the surgical approach, it is critical to remove enough bone, including the subchondral plate on each side of the fusion site, to achieve consistent union rates. One

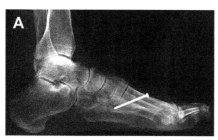
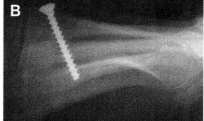

Fig. 4. (*A*) Non–weight-bearing lateral radiograph of a dorsiflexory wedge osteotomy of the first metatarsal with a proximal plantar hinge. The screw is placed from proximal dorsal to distal plantar. (*B*) Weight-bearing lateral radiograph of a dorsiflexory wedge osteotomy of the first metatarsal with a distal plantar hinge. The screw is placed from distal dorsal to proximal plantar.

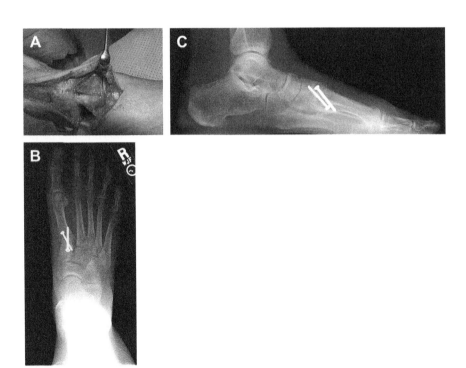

Fig. 5. (A) Intraoperative photograph of a medial approach to the first metatarsocuneiform joint. The access to the joint is facilitated by elevating the soft tissue envelope as a single layer from the joint. (B) Anteroposterior radiograph shows crossed orientation of screw fixation. (C) Lateral radiograph of same patient shows the parallel orientation of the screws.

should realize that resection of the joint causes first ray shortening, although this seldom has clinical consequences.

Fixation of the fusion site is best achieved with lag screws, which are placed in a variety of constructs. The most popular configuration seems to promote delivery of fully threaded cortical screws from the dorsal aspect of the first ray.[14,18] The selected screws are long so that maximal bone is purchased and parallel in the sagittal plane. Delivery of the screws in this fashion is more difficult from a medial approach, such that alternative orientations can be considered. Delivery of a plantar screw from the medial plantar portion of the first metatarsal into the first cuneiform, with a second screw placed from the dorsal first cuneiform provides an inherently stable construct.[19] In particular, this construct is favorable when the support of the subchondral bone plate is absent because of the obligate resection during correction.

Jones Suspension of the First Metatarsal

In the more flexible deformity, the operative strategy can be directed toward reorientation of muscular forces, such that the flexible deformity is "reversed" over time. Transfer of the long extensor tendons directly to the respective metatarsal necks along with interphalangeal fusion was described in tandem as a means to correct the plantar flexed forefoot, primarily in the neuromuscular deprived foot. Specifically, Jones tenosuspension has been contemporized to dorsiflex a mobile first metatarsal and provide stability to the hallux interphalangeal joint by means of fusion. The actual effect of the fusion is to thwart the retrograde plantar flexion force on the first metatarsal head and the resultant supinatory coil of the foot (**Fig. 6**A). This is not to advocate this procedure only in the context of a flexible deformity, however, because it can also maintain a dorsiflexory thrust on the first ray, even if done with repositioning bony procedures. In effect, the tenosuspension helps to rebalance the forces acting on the first metatarsal and prevents relapse.

The operation is performed from a dorsal exposure starting at the interphalangeal joint. The interphalangeal joint is fused with the technique of choice, along with a dorsal release of the first metatarsal phalangeal joint (see **Fig. 6**B). The extensor hallucis longus tendon is carefully removed from its corridor along the dorsal aspect of the first metatarsal all the way back to the metatarsal base in preparation for attachment (see **Fig. 6**C). From a superficial perspective, the dynamic dorsiflexion of the first metatarsal by means of muscular contraction of the extensor hallucis tendon is intriguing.[20] From a mechanical perspective, however, there is far greater mechanical

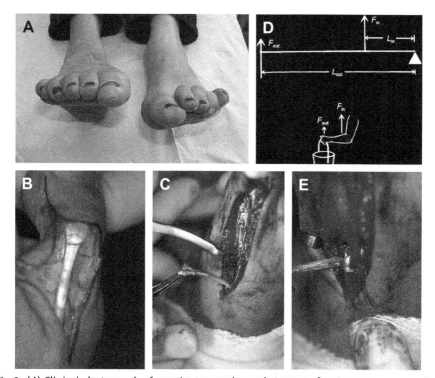

Fig. 6. (A) Clinical photograph of a patient several months' status after Jones tenosuspension and interphalangeal joint fusion on the right foot and preoperative on the left foot. Note the distinction between the feet and the lack of plantar prominence of the first metatarsal head. (B) Intraoperative photograph demonstrates distal exposure. (C) Intraoperative photograph of another patient with the extensor hallucis longus tendon harvested from the sheath and ready for anchoring into the base of the first metatarsal. (D) Diagram depicts the arrangement of a class III lever. Note that as the distance from the rotation point decreases, the mechanical advantage increases. When the extensor hallucis longus is anchored closer to the first metatarsal base, the resultant dorsiflexion force with contraction of the tendon is greater. (E) Photograph shows the long extensor placed through a transverse drill hole in the metatarsal. The tendon is appropriately tensioned and then anchored on itself.

utility when the anchor point of the tendon is closer to the axis of rotation.[21] Whether or not the primary axis of rotation is at the first metatarsal cuneiform joint or not is irrelevant. It is clearly somewhere between the first cuneiform and the talar neck, however. If the long extensor tendon is attached to the distal aspect of the first metatarsal head, as described by Jones,[20] the resultant vector forces create more of an axial load along the long axis of the metatarsal rather than the desired effect of elevation. If the point of tenodesis is close to the metatarsal base, however, the primary vector component is one of dorsiflexion. Essentially, the construct should mimic that of a class III lever (see **Fig. 6**D). The harvested tendon is attached to the base of the metatarsal. It is useful to provide a transversely oriented channel in the base of the metatarsal so that the tension and the actual efficiency of the muscle tendon unit can be modulated. The tendon should be inserted into the lateral side of the first metatarsal base through the bone and adjusted so that proper physiologic tension is attained. The tendon can be sutured on itself or fixated at the desired tension with an interference screw (see **Fig. 6**E). The surgeon should realize that the ankle should be at neutral position during the establishment of the physiologic tension to simulate the net effect of first ray dorsiflexion that occurs during the swing phase of gait.

Adjunctive Procedures

Although beyond the scope of this article, there are several adjunctive procedures that may be required to solidify the surgical approach to this complex deformity. These include plantar fascial releases, hallux interphalangeal joint fusion, peroneal switch, and release of the posterior tibial tendon. It is not easy to assign specific criteria for each of these procedures, but it is difficult to "overcorrect" a cavovarus foot. It is exceedingly rare to regret the performance of too many procedures or overzealous correction of osseous deformities.

Release of the plantar fascia has been described as a necessary component of cavus foot reconstruction.[13,22–24] When the entire forefoot is being mobilized dorsally, in effect, the foot is being lengthened, and an intact plantar fascia may impede the capacity to do so. In most cases, however, it is quite unnecessary to separate the origin of the intrinsic musculature from the calcaneus as a component of this procedure. Even though the digits may plantar flex as the arch height correction is achieved, it is often helpful to reduce the subluxation at the metatarsal phalangeal joints. If persistent and symptomatic digital flexion is evident, local digital procedures are indicated.

Hallux interphalangeal joint surgery is a common procedure in the context of this deformity and has little functional cost to the patient. It is not uncommon to experience lack of hallux purchase after surgical convalescence if the contractures at the first metatarsophalangeal joint are not addressed or recur, however. Practically, some degree of plantar flexion can be incorporated into the fusion mass during the technical execution of the procedure.

The peroneal switch operation involves attachment of the peroneus longus muscle and part of the tendon to the tendon of the peroneus brevis. This effectively converts the longus to an overall pronator of the foot and plantar flexor of the first metatarsal to an everter. Although this benefit is usually subtle at first, over time, the utility of this procedure manifests because removal of the plantar restraint allows the first metatarsal to migrate dorsally.

In summary, complete surgical rehabilitation of the cavoid foot type is predicated on uncoiling of the flexible tripod. Although there is a need to perform hindfoot fusion operations to reduce the height of the arch and rebalance the foot, the impact of the first ray on the morphology and presentation of the cavus foot is weighty. Because of the strategic position of the first ray as the medial pillar of the foot, surgical treatment of the cavoid foot type almost always includes repositioning of the first ray. The effect of these procedures can be realized immediately in the case of bony operations or more slowly in the event that tendon transfers have been used.

REFERENCES

1. Cotton FJ. Foot statics and surgery. N Engl J Med 1936;214:353–62.
2. Paulos L, Coleman SS, Samuelson KM. Pes cavovarus—review of a surgical approach using selective soft tissue procedures. J Bone Joint Surg Am 1980; 62:942–53.
3. Samilson RL, Dillin W. Cavus, cavovarus, and calcaneocavus. Clin Orthop Relat Res 1983;177:125–32.
4. Aminian A, Sangeorzan BJ. The anatomy of cavus foot deformity. Foot Ankle Clin 2008;13:191–8.
5. Hansen ST. The cavovarus/supinated foot deformity and external tibial torsion: the role of the posterior tibial tendon. Foot Ankle Clin 2008;13:325–8.
6. Younger AS, Hansen ST. Adult cavovarus foot. J Am Acad Orthop Surg 2005; 13(5):302–15.
7. Solis G, Hennessy MS, Saxby TS. Pes cavus: a review. Foot Ankle Surg 2000;6: 145–53.
8. McCluskey WP, Lovell MD, Cummings RJ. The cavovarus foot deformity. Clin Orthop Relat Res 1989;247:27–37.
9. Jahss MH. Evaluation of the cavus foot for orthopedic treatment. Clin Orthop Relat Res 1983;181:52–63.
10. Bentzon PGK. Pes cavus and muscular peroneus longus. Acta Orthop Scand 1938;4:50.
11. Coleman S, Chestnut W. A simple test for hindfoot flexibility in the cavovarus foot. Clin Orthop 1977;122:60–2.
12. Jahss MH. Tarsometatarsal truncated-wedge arthrodesis for pes cavus and equinovarus deformity of the fore part of the foot. J Bone Joint Surg Am 1980;62(5): 713–22.
13. Cole WH. The treatment of clawfoot. J Bone Joint Surg Am 1940;22:895–908.
14. Ronald RG, Ching RP, Christensen JC, et al. Biomechanical analysis of the first metatarsocuneiform arthrodesis. J Foot Ankle Surg 1998;37:376–85.
15. Catanzariti AR, Mendicino RW. Technical considerations in tarsometatarsal joint arthrodesis. J Am Podiatr Med Assoc 2005;95(1):85–90.
16. Catanzariti AR, Mendicino RW, Lee MS, et al. The modified Lapidus arthrodesis: a retrospective analysis. J Foot Ankle Surg 1999;38(5):322–32.
17. Patel S, Ford LA, Etcheverry J, et al. Modified Lapidus arthrodesis: rate of nonunion in 227 cases. J Foot Ankle Surg 2004;43(1):37–42.
18. Ray RG. First metatarsocuneiform arthrodesis: technical considerations and technique modification. J Foot Ankle Surg 2002;41:260–72.
19. Schuberth JM. Lapidus procedure, chapter 12. In: Gerbert J, editor. 3rd edition. Textbook of bunion surgery. Philadelphia: WB Saunders; 2001. p. 288–302.
20. Jones R. Claw foot. Brux Med 1916;1:749.
21. Schuberth JM. Tendon transfers. In: Oloff LM, editor. Musculoskeletal disorders of the lower extremities. Philadelphia: WB Saunders; 1994. p. 588–611.
22. Steindler A. Operative treatment of pes cavus. Surg Gynecol Obstet 1917;24:612.
23. Steindler A. Stripping of the os calcis. J Orthop Surg 1920;2:8.
24. Dwyer FC. The present status of the problem of pes cavus. Clin Orthop Relat Res 1975;106.

Procedure Selection for Hallux Valgus

Lawrence A. Ford, DPM, FACFAS[a],*, Graham A. Hamilton, DPM, FACFAS[b]

KEYWORDS

- Hallux valgus • Bunion • Bunionectomy
- Hypermobility • First ray

There are more than 100 different types of surgical procedures described for the correction of hallux valgus deformity.[1,2] It has been the subject of much interest by many foot and ankle surgeons with varying opinions regarding etiology and treatment. For more than a century, a significant portion of the medical literature has focused on bunion surgery, yet there is still much debate and little consensus as to what the best way is to correct this complex and often underappreciated deformity. The criteria for procedure selection for hallux valgus are poorly defined. This has led to high reported failure rates.[3] Clinical studies have supported various procedures based on the successful elimination of pain and bunion deformity. One of the first published treatments of hallux valgus was described by Heuter in 1870 as subcapital amputation of the metatarsal head.[4,5] More than a decade later, Barker described an osteotomy in the metatarsal head that removed a wedge of bone to effectively decompress the bunion.[6] Over the next half a century many modifications were made to this osteotomy to correct the angular malalignment of the first metatarsal and hallux. Hallux valgus surgery has become more sophisticated since its introduction as a "bunionectomy." Focus on reduction of the intermetatarsal angle and other measurable parameters, via osteotomies or fusions, is now the standard of care for bunion "correction". Selecting the appropriate procedure however, is not as straightforward as plugging numbers into a formula. Understanding the biomechanical forces affecting the first ray and the first ray's effects on associated deformity and correlating patient and surgeon goals and expectations are critical factors in determining which procedure is best suited for each patient.

[a] Kaiser San Francisco Bay Area Foot and Ankle Residency Program, Department of Orthopedics and Podiatric Surgery, The Permanente Medical Group, 280 West MacArthur Boulevard, Oakland, CA 94611, USA
[b] Kaiser San Francisco Bay Area Foot and Ankle Residency Program, Department of Orthopedics and Podiatric Surgery, The Permanente Medical Group, 5601 Deer Valley Road, Antioch, CA 94531, USA
* Corresponding author.
E-mail address: lawrence.ford@kp.org (L.A. Ford).

Clin Podiatr Med Surg 26 (2009) 395–407
doi:10.1016/j.cpm.2009.03.005
0891-8422/09/$ – see front matter © 2009 Elsevier Inc. All rights reserved.

podiatric.theclinics.com

FIRST RAY FUNCTION

Historically, the success rate for bunion surgery has not been universally satisfactory, with a high number of patients remaining dissatisfied even when good correction of radiographic measurements was achieved.[7] Many complications have been reported that often parallel the associated morbidities found in patients who have hallux valgus. Plantar callosities, lesser metatarsal stress fractures, second metatarsophalangeal joint (MTPJ) instability, hammertoes, metatarsus elevatus, posterior tibial tendon dysfunction, and other problems can be attributed directly to a dysfunctional first ray with hallux valgus or to complications from hallux valgus surgery (**Fig. 1**).[8–15] Many of these complications are despite excellent correction of the intermetatarsal and hallux abductus angles. King and Toolan warned that this may be due to a failure to recognize or appreciate the implications the first ray has on the proximal foot.[16]

The reliance of the body on normal first ray mechanics strongly suggests that re-establishing normal function of the first ray is of paramount importance. During midstance, a cantilever load is applied to the first ray during normal physiologic loading.[17] It is well known that a structurally stable first ray is necessary for even distribution of weight across the forefoot.[18] When stable and anatomically aligned, the first ray's buttressing effect along the medial column of the foot also resists overpronation of the midfoot and collapse of the medial longitudinal arch.[19] This in turn helps prevent

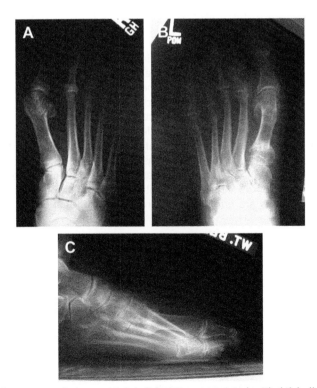

Fig. 1. Second metatarsophalangeal joint dislocation associated with (A) hallux valgus and (B, C) as a consequence of malunion after hallux valgus surgery. As the lesser metatarsal parabola is normal in both cases, it is clear that the lack of proper first ray load sharing has resulted in adjacent metatarsal overload.

medial deflection of body weight and maintains appropriate alignment of the foot with the more proximal joints of the lower extremity. The opposite is true in feet with elevated first rays. Subotnick suggested that forefoot varus is compensated by eversion of the heel until the first ray contacts the ground.[19] The properly functioning first ray provides stability through the windlass mechanism, offering a structurally sound platform during the midstance and propulsive phases of the gait cycle.[20,21] This is especially critical as the leg passes anteriorly over the ankle and the single foot's first ray bears up to one third of the body's weight during late midstance and push off.[11] Girdlestone eloquently stated in 1947 that "the mechanism of the foot is that of a lever of the second order with the fulcrum at the metatarsal heads, and for any system of levers to work efficiently the fulcrum must be stable and the lever rigid."[22] It is easy to see how a dysfunctional first ray, with or without hallux valgus, can deleteriously affect the function of the whole foot and lower extremity. Whether or not the first ray is malaligned, arthritic, hypermobile, long, short, elevated, or unstable, the consequences on the mechanics of the foot can be profound.

Feet with metatarsus primus varus have been shown to carry less than normal loads under the first metatarsal with a subsequent relative increased load under the lesser metatarsals.[18,22–24] A malaligned first metatarsal may adversely affect overall foot function; conversely, a properly aligned first metatarsal can improve alignment of the hindfoot and affect proximal deformity.[25–29] In patients who have hallux valgus and concomitant metatarsalgia, Klaue believes the clinical significance of first ray mobility has been underestimated.[30] The concept of first ray hypermobility is not universally accepted, however, as other studies and opinions have downplayed the causative effects the first ray has on associated foot pathology.[31–33] Coughlin and Jones questioned the existence of hypermobility of the first ray, arguing against its relevance on the rest of the foot. In a thorough review of the literature on hypermobility of the first ray, Roukis and Landsman found that defining this condition is controversial and problematic.[34] As objectively defining hypermobility is elusive, it is difficult to judge its existence or absence. Recognizing that the first ray may not be bearing its fair share of weight is more relevant than the presence or absence of "hypermobility". In normal walking, the greatest loads are found beneath the first metatarsal. The metatarsals must resist bending and shear forces during forefoot loading; otherwise, flattening of the medial longitudinal arch, lesser metatarsal stress fractures, and metatarsalgia may ensue.[18] Yamamoto and colleagues, in evaluating forefoot pressures in patients who had hallux valgus, showed an increase in pressure under the second metatarsal head after a crescentic base osteotomy and McBride bunionectomy despite no significant change in metatarsal length.[24] Regardless of the lack of consensus in scientifically defining hypermobility, it is clear the first ray must bear its appropriate load during midstance and propulsion. If it does not, then it is insufficient and may have profound effects on the rest of the foot. A hypermobile first ray is functionally similar to a short or elevated first ray. Appropriate length, alignment, and stability of the first ray are essential to activation of the windlass mechanism.[21,26] According to Stainsby, restoring first ray function "must surely be one of the main aims of surgery for hallux valgus."[26]

SELECTING THE APPROPRIATE PROCEDURE

The role the first ray plays as an etiologic or aggravating factor in associated foot pathology is important to recognize and address when selecting which procedure is appropriate in the treatment of hallux valgus. Rush stressed the importance of defining the structural contributions and influencing factors that govern the first ray, suggesting that this leads to more accurate procedure selection and subsequently improved functional outcomes.[21] Each procedure for hallux valgus correction is associated with its own inherent potential complications, from delayed union and malunion to overcorrection and recurrence. Although most clinical studies report a higher percentage of successful results than complications, there is no procedure that can successfully apply to all deformities.[35] Most procedures offered in the literature for correction of hallux valgus do work if properly performed in the right indications.[1,36,37] Selecting the proper procedure in the appropriate foot and appropriate patient is the key to the success of each individual procedure. If the right indications are selected, it has been shown that head osteotomies, base osteotomies, and Lapidus arthrodeses have similar rates of complications and need for revision surgery.[38] There are arguments debating first metatarsal head versus base procedures: osteotomies versus Lapidus arthrodesis, soft tissue versus osseous correction, first metatarsophalangeal joint fusion versus arthroplasty, and others. Each procedure has its merits if performed in the right individual and under the right circumstances. Each procedure also will fail if the right indications are not met or the limits of the procedure are pushed too far (Fig. 2). A closing base-wedge osteotomy performed in a short first metatarsal has drastically different results from when it is performed in a long metatarsal. The same can be true for a Keller arthroplasty in active versus sedentary geriatric patients who have an arthritic first MTPJ. Selecting the appropriate procedure for each individual and executing that procedure well are the most important factors in successful hallux valgus surgery.

GOALS AND EXPECTATIONS

A thorough understanding of patient goals and the mechanical influences contributing to a deformity are necessary factors in determining the correct procedure in each individual. In general, anatomic alignment of the intermetatarsal angle and hallux abductus angle, congruency of the joint, anatomic alignment of the sesamoids, first ray length, and function of the windlass mechanism are necessary endpoints if the goal is to create or maintain normal first ray function. If these are not taken into account,

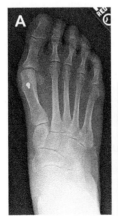
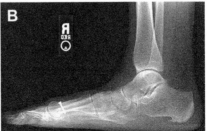

Fig. 2. Recurrent hallux valgus after failed bunionectomy with distal osteotomy (A). The instability of the medial column was not addressed during surgery, as suggested by subluxation at the first tarsometatarsal joint, naviculocuneiform sag, and malalignment of the talar-first metatarsal axis (B).

then the risks for a poor result and dissatisfied patient are much higher. It is a surgeon's duty to understand the goals and expectations of a patient undergoing the proposed surgery. Is the goal to relieve pain with shoe pressure or to relieve pain with walking? If pain occurs only after long hikes or during running, then the expected goals of surgery are different from those for a patient who only may want to wear sensible shoes comfortably. The purpose of understanding the goals of patients is to address these goals and meet the mutual expectations of patients and surgeons.

There are many factors to consider when selecting the appropriate procedure or combination of procedures. The age of patients generally is important but not as valuable as patients' activity level and desired future activity level. Although risk for recurrence is one of the main driving forces behind procedure selection, this may not be given the same level of priority in geriatric patients. The same thought process may apply when considering the ability of the procedure to resist the different forces associated with high-level athletics versus community ambulation. Compromises may be acceptable, or even necessary, at times. The presence or absence of medical comorbidities also plays a role in procedure selection for hallux valgus. Consider a similar severe bunion deformity complicated by pes planovalgus in a young healthy patient and in an elderly patient who had congestive heart failure. Both need to be able to walk without pain to thrive. Although a more aggressive reconstructive operation may be appropriate for fitter and younger patients, a prolonged and more difficult convalescence may be detrimental to unhealthier patients. If the mutual goal is to create or maintain normal first ray function, then it is necessary to obtain good alignment of the first ray and anatomic position of the sesamoids. Selecting the appropriate procedure for each case is not amenable to a protocol or cookbook mentality but should be tailored to the circumstances specific to the goals and expectations of patients and surgeons alike.

ASSOCIATED PATHOLOGY

Important factors in the surgical treatment of hallux valgus include not only correction of the bunion but also the associated pathology caused or aggravated by the bunion deformity. Concomitant pes planovalgus, overpronation of the midfoot, and hypermobility of the first ray have been shown to play an etiologic role in the development of hallux valgus; moreover, their continued presence has been blamed for a higher rate of complications after surgery.[8,16] The first ray is vital to the overall function of the foot and lower extremity, so dysfunction in the form of hallux valgus often is only part of the picture. Hallux valgus can be considered a symptom of a more complicated dysfunctional foot and, if the cause of the symptom is not addressed, then a less than satisfactory outcome may result.

If the issue is indeed isolated hallux valgus in a structurally stable foot, then the treatment is vastly different from that of the foot where the bunion is just one of many symptoms (**Fig. 3**). Concomitant pes planovalgus, lesser metatarsalgia, hammertoes, and hallux limitus are problems often associated with a dysfunctional first ray that complicate the clinical picture. For isolated hallux valgus, the type of procedure performed is not as critical as long as normal length and alignment are maintained. If normal anatomic restraints of weight-bearing distribution are disrupted, then associated pathology can develop as a result of the incorrect bunion procedure. Extra care must be taken in the surgical decision-making process when associated pathology is present. Flat foot deformity not only increases the likelihood of development of hallux valgus but also renders successful correction more difficult. Because overpronation of the midfoot leads to increased medial deflection of body weight, the

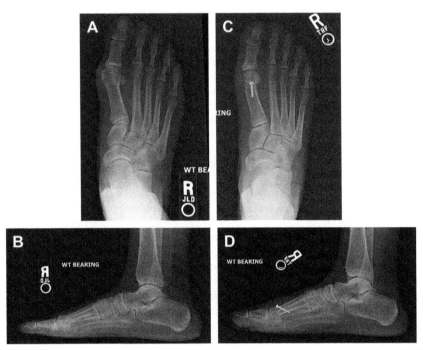

Fig. 3. Pre- and postoperative radiographs of a structurally stable foot with isolated hallux valgus. Because there is no evidence of gross dysfunction of the first ray, a distal osteotomy is appropriate (*A–D*).

biomechanical forces going through the first metatarsal create a bending moment in the medial column. This results in elevation of the first ray and increases the likelihood of recurrence if the first metatarsal cannot act as a stable buttress.[20] A similar scenario ensues if the first metatarsal is congenitally or iatrogenically short, elevated, or hypermobile. In this case, the insufficient first ray can cause collapse of the medial longitudinal arch. Perhaps this is a desired effect in correcting hallux valgus in a cavus foot, but in a normal or flat foot, this only increases dysfunction and deformity.

Lesser metatarsal overload can be secondary to a poorly functioning first ray. Hypermobility has been implicated as a predisposing factor in lesser metatarsalgia. Whether or not the lesser metatarsal symptoms are manifested as pain, synovitis, predislocation syndrome, plantar plate tear, stress fracture, or simply callus, an insufficient first ray can be the cause (**Fig. 4**).[39] Procedure selection, in most cases, is limited to those procedures that address the cause of the lesser metatarsal overload. Stabilizing the first ray is of paramount importance. This does not imply that a Lapidus arthrodesis is necessary to accomplish this. Rush and colleagues demonstrated that reduction of and increased intermetatarsal angle imparts stability to the first ray. They postulated that restoration of anatomic alignment between the first and second metatarsals engages the windlass mechanism, which limits abnormal motion in the first ray.[21] Although increasing the weight-bearing capacity under the first metatarsal head via a Lapidus bunion correction would logically decrease the weight under the adjacent second metatarsal head, this has not been scientifically proven.

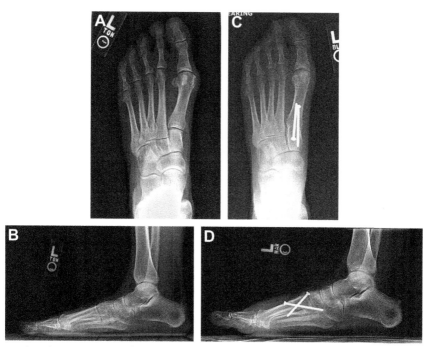

Fig. 4. (*A, B*) A 58-year-old-female who had painful hallux valgus and medial arch pain complicated by instability of the first ray. (*C, D*) A modified Lapidus arthrodesis was performed to stabilize the medial column and provide a buttress of support for the talus. Note the improved alignment at the talonavicular joint on the anteroposterior and lateral projections.

RADIOGRAPHIC ASSESSMENT

Evaluating angular measurements on plain film weight-bearing radiographs of the foot is important in helping select the appropriate procedure for hallux valgus surgery. The severity or size of the deformity has been identified as an important factor in procedure selection. Most studies have relied on clinical satisfaction scores and the analysis of radiographic parameters as means of determining the merits of a particular procedure. Investigation of pre- and postoperative radiographs usually focuses on the intermetatarsal angle, hallux abductus angle, proximal articular set angle (or distal metatarsal angle), and sesamoid position. Although these measurements are important in determining the amount of correction of hallux valgus deformity, they are inadequate determinants of the success of a particular procedure because their effects on overall foot function are not clearly delineated.[16] The focus on radiographic measurements of transverse plane angular deformity of the first metatarsal and hallux has led to its arguably skewed importance in procedure selection. In some cases, emphasis has been placed on intermetatarsal angle correction to such a degree that procedures are pushed past the limits for which they were originally designed.[40,41] The result is a perception that a successful bunion operation is one that simply accomplishes realignment of the first ray in the transverse plane. Although transverse plane correction is important in re-establishing normal mechanics of the first ray, it is by no means sufficient. Sagittal plane, and to a lesser extent frontal plane, realignment also is necessary to restore normal mechanics of the foot. The angular relationship between the first metatarsal and the talus is probably the most important radiographic measurement in assessing stability of the first ray and medial column. Bisection of the talus should run through the first metatarsal head in the anteroposterior and lateral weight-bearing projections. Restoration of this talar-first metatarsal axis helps to re-establish normal anatomic relationships and proper functioning of the first ray. Selecting procedures with this in mind allows surgeons to address the foot as a whole rather than focusing only on the relationship of the first and second metatarsals, hallux, and sesamoids.

Other subjective and objective data are used to help surgeons consider the appropriate surgical procedure for hallux valgus. These include the presence or absence of degenerative changes in the first metatarsophalangeal or tarsometatarsal joint, insufficiency (hypermobility, short length, elevation, and so forth) of the first ray segment, age and activity level of patients, postoperative and rehabilitative considerations, and even cosmesis.

AUTHORS' RELATIVE INDICATIONS
Silver/McBride Bunionectomy

Distal soft tissue realignment for correction of hallux valgus deformity is used primarily in conjunction with osseous correction attained elsewhere in the first ray. It was Silver, however, who popularized the technique of medial capsulorrhaphy, medial exostectomy, and lateral capsular and adductor release.[42] Later, McBride modified this technique by removal of the lateral sesamoid and transfer of the conjoined adductor tendon to the lateral first metatarsal head.[43,44] Mann and Coughlin, after reviewing the results of this procedure in adults, recommended that the fibular sesamoid be preserved because of the high rate of hallux varus after sesamoid excision.[45,46]

Currently, there are few indications for an isolated Silver or McBride bunionectomy. If a surgeon believes the bunion bump pain is purely secondary to hypertrophy of the medial eminence, then a simple "bunionectomy" may be appropriate. Relying on soft tissue balancing to correct osseous angular deformity can lead to a less than satisfactory outcome.

Distal Osteotomy

There are many different types of osteotomies performed in the distal aspect of the first metatarsal to effectively realign the first MTPJ. With the appropriate indications, these can provide excellent correction of the bunion deformity. It was Mitchell and Hawkins and colleagues, however, who described and popularized the technique of a biplanar metaphyseal osteotomy, which achieves lateral and plantar displacement of the capital fragment and shortening of the first metatarsal.[47] Austin initially described the technique for a chevron-type osteotomy of the distal metaphysis of the first metatarsal.[48] With a chevron osteotomy, resection of the medial eminence, distal metatarsal translational osteotomy, and medial capsulorrhaphy are combined to realign the distal first ray, thereby producing some narrowing of the forefoot. Since its initial description, several modifications in the technical part of the procedure have been made, including the angle of the osteotomy and the use of various alternative methods of internal fixation.

Although a relative reduction of the intermetatarsal angle via a distal metatarsal osteotomy can adequately correct deformity and relieve pain, it is less successful in a structurally unstable foot. If the appropriate indications are met, the distal osteotomy can provide excellent long-term correction and relief of pain. If overpronation of the midfoot and insufficiency of the first ray are present, then the risk for recurrence is potentially high, as weight-bearing forces still are directed through the medial forefoot. Pushing the limitations of a distal osteotomy may correct the widened intermetatarsal angle but not necessarily re-establish normal function of the first ray. A distal osteotomy is most successful when the first ray is structurally stable in the absence of rearfoot deformity and central metatarsal overload.

Shaft/Base Osteotomy

Many proximal first metatarsal osteotomies have been described. Because the correction occurs close to the center of rotational angulation (usually at the first tarsometatarsal joint), proximal osteotomies typically have been used for the correction or realignment of large bunion deformities. This is a distinct advantage, allowing for excellent correction of large angular divergence close to the apex of the deformity in the first ray. The disadvantage with these procedures is the technical execution of the osteotomy. There is little room for error with base osteotomies as small degrees of imperfection can result in deleterious effects distally. In advanced hallux valgus without gross instability at the first tarsometatarsal or adjacent joints, shaft and base osteotomies can provide excellent correction. There are many variations. Some techniques describe shortcuts at the base of the metatarsal, such as the proximal chevron and the crescentic osteotomies. Others use long oblique cuts, described as the Ludloff, Juvara, Mau, and Scarf osteotomies. All the procedures have much less intrinsic stability than the distal osteotomies and require more rigid internal fixation and a lengthier postoperative convalescence. Although the distal osteotomies typically can tolerate immediate weight bearing well, most proximal osteotomies require limited to non–weight bearing for approximately 4 to 6 weeks. These procedures generally heal well and nonunion rates are low. Therefore, base osteotomies in particular are useful procedures in patients who smoke tobacco because osteotomies in metaphyseal bone are less likely to result in nonunion than shaft osteotomies or fusions. One of the major complications with base osteotomies is dorsal malunion, most likely due to premature weight bearing or plastic deformation.

Lapidus Arthrodesis

The Lapidus arthrodesis is a powerful tool for the correction of hallux valgus as it attempts to address the deformity at its apex. Its main disadvantages are the potential for nonunion and the recommendation for prolonged non–weight bearing postoperatively. Its advantages are severalfold, most notably its ability to positively affect hindfoot malalignment and offload the central forefoot. Arthrodesis of the first tarsometatarsal joint in conjunction with a distal soft tissue procedure for correction of hallux valgus was popularized by Lapidus, although it was conceived by Albrecht, Kleinberg, and Truslow.[49–52] The procedure is predicated on the principle that metatarsus primus varus must be corrected to obtain satisfactory correction of the hallux valgus deformity. Initially, Lapidus specified that a suitable patient preferably should be "young and robust," with an intermetatarsal angle of 15° or greater and a "fixed" deformity of the first tarsometatarsal joint. Recently, the Lapidus has been advocated for hallux valgus with a hypermobile first ray. Although agreement in defining hypermobility and instability of the first ray remains elusive, the main indications for a Lapidus are hallux valgus with concomitant symptoms related to insufficiency of the medial column of the foot. In the presence of flatfoot deformity or signs of lesser metatarsal overload, it has been believed that arthrodesis at the first tarsometatarsal joint can effectively address these problems by increasing the weight-bearing load under the first metatarsal.

First Metatarsophalangeal Joint Fusion

Arthrodesis of the first MTPJ is useful as a primary procedure to correct severe or geriatric hallux valgus deformity, hallux valgus with rheumatoid arthritis, hallux rigidus, or traumatic arthritis. It also can be useful as a salvage procedure for failed bunion surgery or previous infection.[53,54] Extensively studied in the rheumatoid forefoot, fusion of the first MTPJ also can be an excellent procedure in nonrheumatoid patients.

Its main usefulness is in the presence of arthritis but it also can be effective for severe deformity and in geriatric patients. Although joint motion is sacrificed, the preservation of stability usually allows for unhindered return to most activities. Furthermore, fusion of the great toe joint can reduce large angular deformity between the first and second metatarsals without need for a proximal osteotomy. Perhaps because the lever arm of the first ray is extended, fusion of the first MTPJ also has the ability to decrease the amount of pressure under the central metatarsals.

Keller Bunionectomy

Riedel, in 1886, was the first to perform a resection of the base of the proximal phalanx and arthroplasty of the MTPJ as treatment of hallux valgus.[55] The purpose of the procedure in the treatment of hallux valgus is to decompress the MTPJ by resection of approximately a third of the proximal phalanx, thereby relaxing the contracted lateral structures. Although the Keller procedure probably was once the most widely used bunion procedure, with the development of other surgical techniques and critical clinical evaluation of results of the Keller procedure, its limitations and indications are now better defined.

Keller arthroplasty of the first MTPJ usually is reserved for the inactive geriatric patients who have severe pain in the joint secondary to hallux valgus or arthritis. Although it is effective in relieving pain and deformity, the loss of intrinsic stability to the joint renders the first ray dysfunctional. The most common consequence is painful transfer overload of the lesser metatarsals.

Implant Arthroplasty

The use of a MTPJ prosthesis in primary bunion surgery rarely is indicated. The occasional sedentary patients who have advanced MTPJ degenerative arthritis and who desire a prosthesis may be candidates for the procedure. As with a Keller bunionectomy, the major disadvantage of most implant bunionectomies is the loss of intrinsic stability to the joint. The advantage over a Keller is the ability of the implant to provide a physical spacer that more predictably holds the joint in anatomic position. Because the tendoligamentous attachments around the first MTPJ are sacrificed, the first ray is not able to adequately support forefoot loading and propulsion.

Akin Osteotomy

The primary indication for this procedure is a hallux valgus interphalangeus deformity.[56] A typical Akin procedure achieves correction of hallux valgus deformity by means of a medial closing wedge osteotomy in the proximal phalanx.[57] This procedure can produce a satisfactory result in the treatment of specific types of deformities but is not indicated in the presence of MTPJ subluxation. The Akin-type osteotomy in the proximal phalanx of the hallux is used primarily to straighten the great toe. When combined metatarsal correction and soft tissue balancing are not sufficient, the Akin can improve the alignment of the first MTPJ.

SUMMARY

Correcting pain and deformity, avoiding recurrence, and preserving or establishing normal foot function are the ultimate goals of hallux valgus surgery. Rather than choosing procedures based on the degree of the intermetatarsal angle, a more logical approach is to attempt to restore normal mechanics of the first ray, for which angular correction is only one consideration. A successful outcome is dependent on selecting the appropriate procedure and executing it well.

REFERENCES

1. Coetzee JC, Resig SG, Kuskowski M, et al. The Lapidus procedure as salvage after failed surgical treatment of hallux valgus: a prospective cohort study. J Bone Joint Surg Am 2003;85-A:60–5.
2. Kelikian, Hampar. Hallux valgus, allied deformities of the forefoot and metatarsalgia. Philadelphia: WB Saunders; 1965.
3. Scranton PE. Principles in bunion surgery: current concepts review. J Bone Joint Surg Am 1983;65(7):1026–28.
4. Heuter C. Klinik der Gelenkkrankheiten mit Einschluss der Orthopadie. Leipzig: FCW Vogel; 1870–71. (Quoted by Glynn, JBJS 62-B(2):188–91, 1980).
5. Glynn MK, Dunlop JB, Fitzpatrick D. The Mitchell distal metatarsal osteotomy for hallux valgus. J Bone Joint Surg Am 1980;62-B(2):188–91.
6. Barker AE. An operation for hallux valgus. Lancet 1884;1:655.
7. Ferrari J, Higgins JP, Williams RL. Interventions for treating hallux valgus (abductovalgus) and bunions. Cochrane Database Syst Rev 2000;(2):CD000964.
8. Roling BA, Christensen JC, Johnson CJ. Biomechanics of the first ray. Part IV: the effect of selected medial column arthrodeses. A three-dimensional kinematic analysis in a cadaver model. J Foot Ankle Surg 2002;41(5):278–85.
9. Meyer JM, Tomeno B, Burdet A. Metatarsalgia due to insufficient support by the first ray. Int Orthop 1981;5:193–201.
10. Bevilacqua NJ, Rogers LC, Wrobel JS, et al. Restoration and preservation of first metatarsal length using the distraction Scarf osteotomy. J Foot Ankle Surg 2008; 47(2):96–102.
11. Viladot A. Metatarsalgia due to biomechanical alterations of the forefoot. Orthop Clin North Am 1973;41:165–78.
12. Bolland BJ, Sauve PS, Taylor GR. Rheumatoid forefoot reconstruction: first metatarsophalangeal joint fusion combined with Weil's metatarsal osteotomies of the lesser rays. J Foot Ankle Surg 2008;47(2):80–8.
13. Mann RA, Thompson FM. Arthrodesis of the first metatarsophalangeal joint for hallux valgus in rheumatoid arthritis. J Bone Joint Surg Am 1984;66:687–92.
14. Bouche RT, Heit EJ. Combined plantar plate and hammertoe repair with flexor digitorum longus tendon transfer for chronic, severe sagittal plane instability of the lesser metatarsophalangeal joints: preliminary observations. J Foot Ankle Surg 2008;47(2):125–37.
15. Vianna VF, Myerson MS. Complications of hallux valgus surgery. Management of the short first metatarsal and the failed resection arthroplasty. Foot Ankle Clin 1998;3(1):33–49.
16. King DM, Toolan BC. Associated deformities and hypermobility in hallux valgus: an investigation with weightbearing radiographs. Foot Ankle Int 2004;25(4): 251–5.
17. Ray RG, Ching RP, Christensen JC, et al. Biomechanical analysis of the first metatarsocuneiform arthrodesis. J Foot Ankle Surg 1998;37(5):376–85.

18. Stokes IAF, Hutton WC, Stott JRR. Forces acting on the metatarsals during normal walking. J Anat 1979;129(3):579–90.
19. Subotnick S. The flat foot. Phys Sportsmed 1981;9(8):85–91.
20. Johnson CJ, Christensen JC. Biomechanics of the first ray. Part I: the effects of peroneus longus function: a three-dimensional kinematic study on a cadaver model. J Foot Ankle Surg 1999;38(5):313–21.
21. Rush SM, Christensen JC, Johnson CJ. Biomechanics of the first ray. Part II: metatarsus primus varus as a cause of hypermobility. A three-dimensional kinematic analysis in a cadaver model. J Foot Ankle Surg 2000;39(2):68–77.
22. Girdlestone GR. Physiotherapy for hand and foot. Physiotherapy for hand and foot 1947;9:167–9.
23. Stokes IAF, Hutton WC, Evans MJ. The effects of hallux valgus and Keller's operation on the load-bearing function of the foot during walking. Acta Orthop Belg 1975;41:695–704.
24. Yamamoto H, Muneta T, Asahina S, et al. Forefoot pressures during walking in feet afflicted with hallux valgus. Clin Orthop Relat Res 1996;323:247–53.
25. Bojsen-Moller F. Anatomy of the forefoot, normal and pathologic. Clin Orthop Relat Res 1978;142:10–8.
26. Stainsby GD. Pathologic anatomy and dynamic effect of the displaced plantar plate and the importance of the integrity of the plantar plate-deep transverse metatarsal ligament tie-bar. Ann R Coll Surg Engl 1997;79:58–68.
27. Avino A, Patel S, Hamilton GA, et al. The effect of the Lapidus arthrodesis on the medial longitudinal arch: a radiographic review. J Foot Ankle Surg 2008;47(6):510–4.
28. Cameron HU, Fedorkow DM. Revision rates in forefoot surgery. Foot Ankle Int 1982;3(1):47–9.
29. Hedrick MR. The plantar aponeurosis: current topic review. Foot Ankle Int 1996; 17(10):646–9.
30. Klaue K, Hansen ST, Masquelet AC. Clinical, quantitative assessment of first tarsometatarsal mobility in the sagittal plane and its relation to hallux valgus deformity. Foot Ankle Int 1994;15(1):9–13.
31. Coughlin MJ, Jones CP. Hallux valgus and first ray mobility. A prospective study. J Bone Joint Surg Am 2007;89(9):1887–98.
32. Grebing BR, Coughlin MJ. Evaluation of Morton's theory of second metatarsal hypertrophy. J Bone Joint Surg Am 2004;86(7):1375–86.
33. Glasoe WM, Coughlin MJ. A critical analysis of Dudley Morton's concept of disordered foot function. J Foot Ankle Surg 2006;45(3):147–55.
34. Roukis TS, Landsman AS. Hypermobility of the first ray: a critical review of the literature. J Foot Ankle Surg 2003;42(6):377–90.
35. Williams L, Wilson S, Kuwada G. A comprehensive retrospective analysis of complications and radiographic findings following bunionectomy procedures for first ray deformities. Lower Extremity 1995;2(1):11–28.
36. Kitaoka HB, Patzer GL. Salvage treatment of failed hallux valgus operations with proximal first metatarsal osteotomy and distal soft tissue reconstruction. Foot Ankle Int 1998;19(3):127–31.
37. Haas Z, Hamilton G, Sundstrom D, et al. Maintenance of correction of first metatarsal closing base wedge osteotomies versus modified Lapidus arthrodesis for moderate to severe hallux valgus deformity. J Foot Ankle Surg 2007;46(5): 358–65.
38. Lagaay PM, Hamilton GA, Ford LA, et al. Rates of revision surgery using chevron-Austin osteotomy, Lapidus arthrodesis, and closing base wedge osteotomy for correction of hallux valgus deformity. J Foot Ankle Surg 2008;47(4):267–72.

39. Hansen ST. Functional Reconstruction of the Foot and Ankle. Philadelphia, PA: Lippincott Williams and Wilkins; 2000. p. 28–9.
40. Stienstra JJ, Lee JA, Nakadate DT. Large displacement distal chevron osteotomy for the correction of hallux valgus deformity. J Foot Ankle Surg 2002;41(4): 213–20.
41. Murawski DE, Beskin JL. Increased displacement maximizes the utility of the distal chevron osteotomy for hallux valgus deformity correction. Foot Ankle Int 2008;29(2):155–63.
42. Silver D. The operative treatment of hallux valgus. J Bone Joint Surg Am 1923;5: 225–32.
43. McBride ED. A conservative operation for bunions. J Bone Joint Surg Am 1928; 10:735–9.
44. McBride ED. A conservative operation for "bunions": end results and refinements of technique. JAMA 1935;105:1164–8.
45. Mann RA, Coughlin MJ. Hallux valgus—etiology, anatomy, treatment and surgical considerations. Clin Orthop Relat Res 1981;157(31):31–41.
46. Mann RA, Pfeffinger L. Hallux valgus repair. DuVries modified McBride procedure. Clin Orthop Relat Res 1991;272:213–8.
47. Hawkins F, Mitchell C, Hedrick D. Correction of hallux valgus by metatarsal osteotomy. J Bone Joint Surg Am 1945;37:387–94.
48. Lapidus PW. Operative treatment of metatarsus primus varus in hallux valgus. Surg Gynecol Obstet 1934;58:183–91.
49. Austin DW, Leventon EO. A new osteotomy for hallux valgus: a horizontally directed "V" displacement osteotomy of the metatarsal head for hallux valgus and primus varus. Clin Orthop 1981;157:25–30.
50. Albrecht G. The pathology and treatment of hallux valgus. Russk Vrach 1911;10: 14–9.
51. Kleinberg S. Operative cure of hallux valgus and bunions. Am J Surg 1932;15: 75–81.
52. Truslow W. Metatarsus primus varus or hallux valgus? J Bone Joint Surg Am 1925; 7:98–108.
53. Coughlin MJ, Grebing BR, Jones CP. Arthrodesis of the metatarsophalangeal joint for idiopathic hallux valgus: intermediate results. Foot Ankle Int 2005;26: 783–92.
54. Tourne Y, Saragaglia D, Zattara A, et al. Hallux valgus in the elderly: metatarsophalangeal arthrodesis of the first ray. Foot Ankle Int 1997;18:195–8.
55. Riedel HL. Zur operativen Behandlung des Hallux valgus. Zentralbl Chir 1886;44: 573–80.
56. Plattner PF, Van Manen JW. Results of Akin type proximal phalangeal osteotomy for correction of hallux valgus deformity. Orthopedics 1990;13:989–96.
57. Akin O. The treatment of hallux valgus: a new operative procedure and its results. Med Sentinel 1925;33:678–9.

Metatarsus Primus Varus Correction: The Osteotomies

Matthew D. Sorensen, DPM, FACFAS[a], Christopher F. Hyer, DPM, FACFAS[a],*

KEYWORDS

- Metatarsis primus varus • Hallux valgus
- Hypermobility • Distal first metatarsal osteotomy
- Proximal metatarsal osteotomy • Lapidus • Correction
- Apex of deformity

Both podiatric and orthopedic surgeons treat hallux valgus. Approximately 33% of individuals in shod populations have some degree of hallux valgus[1] and over 200,000 hallux valgus operations are performed in the United States each year.[2] The deformity itself varies from mild to severe (**Fig. 1**). The literature describes numerous operative procedures for this common malady. The etiology and best operative treatment, however, remain controversial. This article first reviews the utility of first-metatarsal osteotomies in the correction of hallux valgus or metatarsus primus varus, and then demonstrates the effectiveness of first-metatarsal osteotomies in restoring stable mechanics of the first ray without the need for arthrodesis.

Many reports in the literature suggest the Lapidus procedure, or first-tarsometatarsal fusion, is the only procedure to adequately address bunion with a moderate or larger intermetatarsal angle secondary to the "atavistic" relationship between first-ray hypermobility and hallux valgus formation. Proximal metatarsal osteotomies are often indicated for mild, moderate, and severe hallux valgus deformities. Several recent published studies have suggested that realignment of the first ray through osteotomy in the appropriately selected patient may negate the need for first-metatarsal–cuneiform fusion. Hypermobility or instability of the first ray can often be adequately stabilized by realignment of the bone and soft tissue structures. This allows the effects of the windlass mechanism of the plantar fascia, as well as the stabilizing force of the peroneus longus, to be reestablished without sacrifice of the first tarsometatarsal joint.

HISTORY

Surgical intervention for hallux valgus dates back at least to Gernet in 1836. Nineteenth-century physicians surmised the notion of structural change for hallux valgus.

[a] Advanced Foot and Ankle Surgery Fellowship, Orthopedic Foot and Ankle Center, 300 Polaris Parkway, Suite 2000, Westerville, OH 43082, USA
* Corresponding author.
E-mail address: cfh_ofa@yahoo.com (C.F. Hyer).

Clin Podiatr Med Surg 26 (2009) 409–425
doi:10.1016/j.cpm.2009.03.007
0891-8422/09/$ – see front matter © 2009 Elsevier Inc. All rights reserved.

podiatric.theclinics.com

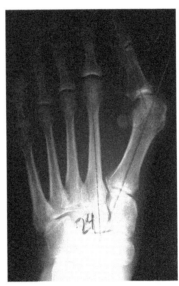

Fig.1. Dorsal-plantar radiograph of weight-bearing left foot shows severe hallux valgus with primus metatarsus varus deformity.

Their efforts led to the introduction of the Reverdin osteotomy[3] in 1881 and to others, such as the Mayo,[4] the Keller,[5] and the Brandes.[6]

The evolution of modern-day operative treatment for hallux valgus has journeyed through innumerable biomechanical, genetic, traumatic, and idiopathic etiologic theories. It seems in recent years, the gestalt of surgical intervention of hallux valgus has teetered between two dominating theories, one based on biomechanics and the other based on clinical study. Without a single unifying theory on which to base surgical intervention, foot and ankle surgeons have formed their own opinions regarding their procedure selection and ideology.

The active debate centers at first metatarsocuneiform joint fusion versus metatarsal osteotomy for surgical intervention of hallux valgus and stabilization of the first ray. Each camp has sound biomechanical, theoretical, and clinical research to support one over the other. This article examines the argument for osteotomy with distal soft tissue release (DSTR).

INDICATIONS

Indications for surgical intervention include a symptomatic clinical and radiographic hallux valgus deformity. Before surgical intervention, exhaustion of conservation care is recommended, including, but not limited to, ice, rest, accommodative padding, nonsteroidal anti-inflammatory drug therapy, orthoses, splinting, physical therapy, and shoe-gear modification. Upon failure of conservative measures, surgical intervention can be considered in the appropriately selected patient.

Comorbidities, such as diabetes mellitus, rheumatoid arthritis, peripheral neuropathy, tobacco or drug abuse, and history of blood clot or hematologic disorder, among others, need to be carefully considered. Also, the social support structure and work environment are important considerations when making the decision for or against surgical intervention. The patient should clearly understand the postoperative course, expected outcomes, and potential complications and risks before going forward.

PROCEDURE SELECTION

There is a general consensus that many factors figure into the selection of corrective surgery for a particular bunion deformity. This decision is partly based on the degree and severity of deformity, the involvement of soft tissue and bone malalignment, and the surgeon's expertise and comfort with certain procedures. Most surgeons agree that for a "mild" deformity, a distal osteotomy is appropriate and provides reliable correction. It is in cases of moderate to severe deformity where surgeons seem to have varied opinions about procedures involving osteotomies of the diaphysis or base of the first metatarsal. The necessity of moving the correction more proximal is based on the simple mathematical/physical understanding of deformity.

DISTAL OSTEOTOMIES

Distal osteotomy in the treatment of hallux valgus deformity is generally reserved for first-second intermetatarsal angles of lesser magnitude with the upper limit generally noted at 14° to 15°. Originators of distal osteotomies have recommended no more than 25% to 50% translation of the distal fragment in relation to the metatarsal shaft.[7–12] Geometric and physical analysis has shown that the 25% to 50% magnitude of capital fragment lateral displacement lacks the ability to correct moderate to large first-second intermetatarsal angles.[13–16]

Other factors to consider in the decision for distal osteotomy correction include the presence of metatarsus adductus or skewfoot deformity, as well as any hindfoot valgus deformity, which places the apex of the deformity much farther proximal and may render a distal osteotomy inadequate.

Following reports by Austin and colleagues,[7,17] the chevron osteotomy has become widely accepted for the correction of mild to moderate hallux valgus deformity. The "V" shape of the osteotomy is thought to provide inherent stability with the ability of the capital fragment to impact upon the shaft of the metatarsal after translation. This quality aides in the strength of the construct. In fact, some purport the lack in need for fixation due to this stability. That being said, subsequent investigators have noted more loss of correction or avascular necrosis in chevron bunionectomies performed without fixation.[15,18] Muhlbauer[19] performed a prospective study using k-wire fixation for the chevron bunionectomy in 55 feet. At an average follow-up of 34 months, there was no case of metatarsal head displacement or loss of correction. Foot and ankle surgeons today generally favor the use of fixation as an aid for stability and report overall satisfaction among patients and surgeons with the procedure.

Generally, the procedure can be performed on an outpatient basis under local/ minimal anesthetic concentration anesthesia, with or without a tourniquet. Per surgeon preference, the patient can be casted or placed into a soft dressing with stiff-soled walking shoe. One of the "selling points" of a distal procedure is the ability to maintain the patient on partial weight-bearing immediately after surgical intervention with weight placed back on the heel until adequate bone healing is noted on radiographs. Early weight-bearing decreases the morbidity, overall recovery time, and chances of deep vein thrombosis. Patients also appreciate the freedom weight-bearing mobility offers them.

As stated, the distal osteotomies have a role in mild deformity correction but are limited because they are distal. The lever arm in correction is short and thus limited to the lesser deformity (**Fig. 2**). As the point of deformity correction moves more proximal, larger degrees of deformity can be addressed.

MIDSHAFT OSTEOTOMY

Virtually any metatarsal osteotomy can be performed in the diaphyseal shaft and subsequently retain the label of midshaft osteotomy. The scarf osteotomy and the "long-arm" chevron osteotomy have gained popularity in recent years secondary to their inherent stability. Weil, Gudas,[20] and Zygmunt[21] began to popularize the scarf in the early 1980s, and Barouk[22] took the osteotomy to Europe in the early 1990s. A number of modifications to the scarf have been described including the short scarf, the long scarf, and the inverted scarf.[22–25]

The interlocking scarf has been used for centuries as a carpentry principle. Its primary contribution is its inherent stability and ability to distribute load. Orthopedically, it initially appeared it would be the panacea for addressing complex issues of strength, stability, and ability to correct a wider range of intermetatarsal angles. The osteotomy is also amenable to single- or multiscrew fixation.

However, reports have indicated that the scarf is not without complications.[26] Also, the assertion that it could correct a larger intermetatarsal angles is being debated widely.[27] The distal and proximal vertical arms of the osteotomy should be limited to 2 to 3 mm in depth to avoid the stress riser into the dorsal/plantar cortex and to decrease the incidence and magnitude of "troughing."[28]

The troughing phenomenon is more frequent in the short scarf secondary to the proximal arm location in the less compact diaphyseal medullary bone, while the distal segment remains in the more compact metaphyseal metatarsal head. This is reportedly more limited in the long scarf as both arms are located within metaphyseal bone.[20] In addition, with the more shallow distal and proximal arms, the amount of

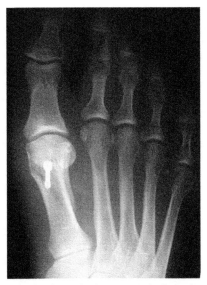

Fig. 2. Dorsal-plantar radiograph of weight-bearing right foot shows mild deformity correction accomplished with distal osteotomy.

troughing is limited to the depth of these vertical cuts.[28] It should be noted, however, that troughing still occurs rather frequently using the long-arm scarf with subsequent elevation of the first ray and impending sequelae. Also, to perform the long-arm osteotomy, substantially greater amounts of periosteal stripping are required, further increasing the incidence and risk of avascular necrosis.

Two-plane correction can be obtained with the scarf during lateral translation of the capital fragment by orienting the horizontal cut plantarly or dorsally. In addition, lengthening and shortening (by removing equal segments of the short arms) of the metatarsal can be retained using the scarf.[28]

Attempts to convert the scarf into a three-plane correctional osteotomy have also been reported. These attempts include one to distract the capital fragment and rotate it in the transverse plane upon lateral translation. This rotation would theoretically enable the osteotomy to act more as a transverse plane rotational metatarsal base procedure for increasingly larger intermetatarsal angles. This conversion attempt is inappropriate for this truly translational osteotomy, however, because the attempted rotation (1) undermines the inherent stability of the scarf, (2) can introduce a coronal plane troughing element with subsequent shortening of the first ray, and (3) can make fixation more of a challenge.

In a study by Deenik[29] comparing the corrective capacities of the distal chevron versus the scarf in hallux valgus treatment, investigators found, against their hypothesis, that the lateral translation in both osteotomies was the same. Because bony contact is essential for adequate fixation, the limiting factor in lateral translation becomes the width of the metatarsal head. Moreover, they found that the corrected metatarsal head, not the shape of the metatarsal shaft, defines the biomechanical axis and, therefore, the intermetatarsal angle.[30] Subsequently, the investigators concluded in favor of the chevron osteotomy over the scarf because the procedure is technically less demanding.

Other more effective and predictable rotational osteotomies are available when the desire is larger intermetatarsal correction. Lack of technical comfort with other procedures is an ill-advised indication for pushing the limits of the scarf. Thus, many investigators agree that the scarf has no greater indication than a distal osteotomy regarding the magnitude of transverse plane correction.[27] The scarf remains a viable procedure for mild to moderate bunion deformities. The modifications presented here are meant to guide the surgeon in attempts to set some level of expectation as well to limit complication.

PROXIMAL METATARSAL OSTEOTOMIES

As a general principle, the severity of the hallux valgus deformity dictates treatment options. The need for metatarsal base osteotomies arises upon encountering patients with first-second intermetatarsal angles of greater magnitude, with the spectrum threshold of around 13° to 15° and greater.[31] The available degree of correction in the proximal osteotomy is substantially greater than that for distal or midshaft osteotomies, given the more proximal location of the axis of rotation.

In the early twentieth century, Loison and colleagues[32–34] reported on their experience with proximal osteotomies. Several proximal osteotomies have been reported to yield good clinical results, including osteotomies involving the proximal chevron, closing and opening base wedges, the Ludloff procedure, the crescentic procedure, and the Mau procedure.[31,35–45]

The proximal crescentic procedure, as popularized by Mann,[41] is the only osteotomy of this kind that requires a crescentic saw blade. The proposed benefits include a truly rotational osteotomy with ability to correct in all three planes with minimal shortening. The long-standing concerns, however, are its inherent lack of stability and subsequent complication of dorsiflexion malunion, as well as difficulty in fixation.[37,41,45–47]

Several studies have compared the crescentic to other proximal osteotomies. A prospective randomized comparison (level II evidence) of the proximal crescentic versus the proximal chevron denoted favorable radiographic correction and clinical outcomes for both. However, dorsiflexion malunion was observed in 17% of the proximal crescentic osteotomies (**Fig. 3**).[48]

A level II evidentiary study by Hyer and colleagues[30] compared the crescentic and Mau osteotomies. Satisfactory correction was noted in both groups and no statistical difference was seen in the magnitude of correction between the two. Statistical differences were noted between the crescentic and Mau in regards to complications. Transarticular hardware positioned in the first tarsometatarsal joint occurred in 40% of crescentic osteotomy cases. The nonunion rate was 50% in the crescentic group and only 4.2% in the Mau group. The investigators did relate, however, that given a longer period for follow-up the union rate may have increased for the crescentic. They concluded that given the amount of correction achieved using the Mau, and its lower incidence of postoperative complications, they prefer it to the crescentic for correction of moderate to severe hallux valgus.

In one of the original articles describing the procedure, Mann noted dorsiflexion malunions in 28% of cases.[41] Numerous investigators have made modifications to the crescentic in attempts to aid overall stability. Jones[48] described a technique orienting the saw blade correctly in the coronal plane to minimize the risk of initial dorsiflexion malpositioning. Perhaps the most logical modification to the crescentic osteotomy itself was the one suggested by Cohen.[49] This modification uses a plantar shelf exiting distal to the osteotomy, thus imparting more stability to the cut as well as ease of fixation.

The advent of foot-specific locked plating may lead to decreased incidence of dorsal malunion for all proximal osteotomies, including that seen in the crescentic. A study by Gallentine[50] concluded a locked plate construct held alignment and position of the proximal chevron first-ray osteotomy without clinical evidence of transfer lesion or hardware-related symptoms. In the authors' recent experience, locked plating has greatly facilitated success toward correction with the crescentic osteotomy. The robust nature of the locked plating systems largely eliminates the incidence of dorsal malunion or any instability secondary to the inherence of the osteotomy construct. Also, by eliminating the need for interfragmentary screw placement, locked

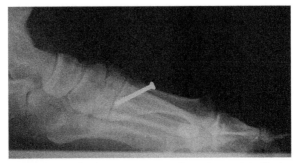

Fig. 3. Lateral radiograph of weight-bearing right foot shows dorsiflexion malunion after proximal crescentic osteotomy.

plating diminishes the possibility of inadvertent intra-articular screw placement. In context, however, again because of the disarticulated and unstable nature of this bone cut, a significant degree of difficulty in initial correction on the table can be encountered with the crescentic.

The Mau osteotomy of the proximal first metatarsal is another procedure used for the correction of moderate-to-severe hallux valgus (**Fig. 4**). It entails the use of a through-and-through, transverse plane osteotomy that extends plantar-proximal to dorsal-distal and has been referred to as a reverse Ludloff osteotomy.[43,44] It has tri-planar correction capacity. Mau, it is said, questioned the stability of the Ludloff osteotomy and used the dorsal shelf to resist the potentially disruptive forces of weight bearing.[44] Although early use of both the Ludloff and Mau osteotomies did not involve internal fixation, more recent reports of these procedures describe the use of osteosynthesis techniques to minimize the risk of complication related to bone healing.[44,51] Moreover, the Mau osteotomy, because of the presence of a dorsal shelf to resist dorsal displacement forces, may impart superior intrinsic stability in comparison to other proximal osteotomies.[30]

In an evaluation of the relative fatigue strength (load to failure) of the Mau, Ludloff, and crescentic osteotomies, Acevedo and colleagues[52] reported that the Mau and Ludloff osteotomies, in comparison to the crescentic osteotomy, were more resistant to fatigue failure. In a comparison of six cadaveric first-metatarsal shaft osteotomies, the Mau osteotomy was shown to be statistically significantly superior in strength and stiffness compared with all other osteotomies except the Ludloff.[51]

The Ludloff osteotomy was introduced in 1913 but failed to gain acceptance because the original description did not include fixation.[53] The advent of screw fixation brought about new interest in the procedure.[39] The Ludloff osteotomy is oriented from proximal-dorsal to distal-plantar and can be oriented in the sagittal plane so as to influence dorsiflexion or plantarflexion upon translation/rotation in the transverse plane, thus allowing correction in all three planes. Upon fixation, the first screw is placed

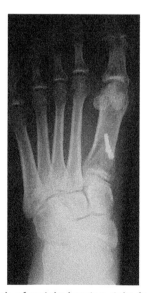

Fig. 4. Dorsal-plantar radiograph of weight-bearing right foot shows successful correction with Mau osteotomy in proximal metatarsal.

before the osteotomy is completed, allowing the surgeon to maintain full control of the osteotomy throughout the procedure.[39] A number of recent clinical series (level IV evidence) have analyzed the modified Ludloff in combination with a distal soft tissue procedure. Trnka[54] related favorable outcome results on the largest cohort of patients known to date having undergone the Ludloff. The mean American Orthopaedic Foot and Ankle Score (AOFAS) improved to 88 points from 53 points at 34-month follow-up. The mean hallux valgus angle decreased significantly from 35° preoperatively to 9° at the most recent follow-up, and the mean intermetatarsal angle decreased significantly to 8° from 17°. All osteotomy sites united without dorsiflexion malunion, but did have a mean first-metatarsal shortening of 2.2 mm.

The authors would also assert that the Mau and Ludloff osteotomies are less difficult to perform and can be learned more quickly than the crescentic osteotomy. This makes for fewer inadvertant or operator-related postoperative sequelae.

The opening wedge proximal metatarsal osteotomy, initially described by Trethowan in 1923, did not gain early acceptance because of lack of adequate fixation and corrective maintenance.[34] With the advent of fixed-angle wedge plates and locked plating, the procedure has become more viable in recent years. Bone graft—either autograft, allograft, or bone substitute—is generally required to fill the gap left by the opening wedge. The benefit of the opening wedge is maintenance of length, which can be necessary in those patients with a short first metatarsal. There has been, to date, no evidence demonstrating that the opening wedge elongates the metatarsal. In addition, this osteotomy can also correct deformity in three planes by orienting the axis/hinge of the osteotomy in the coronal and sagittal planes (**Figs. 5** and **6**).

The closing base wedge osteotomy is similar to the opening wedge osteotomy. However, with the closing base wedge osteotomy, the hinge is maintained on the medial metatarsal cortex and a wedge of bone removed. Reports have described the wedge being removed in an orientation perpendicular to the metatarsal long

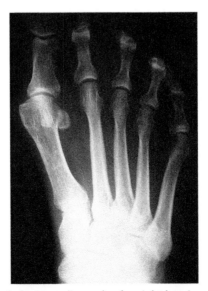

Fig. 5. Preoperative dorsal-plantar radiograph of weight-bearing right foot demonstrates moderate hallux valgus deformity with widening of the first-second intermetatarsal angle.

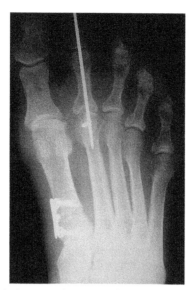

Fig. 6. Postoperative dorsal-plantar radiograph of weight-bearing right foot shows correction via proximal opening wedge osteotomy with plate fixation.

axis as well as oblique to the metatarsal long axis. The oblique closing wedge is more amenable to two-screw fixation. Also, because the apex/hinge is theoretically stronger when placed in the proximal medial–most corner of the first metatarsal, an oblique closing wedge is theoretically more stable. Skepticism has been encountered with this osteotomy based on reports of dorsiflexion malunion, as well as "shortening."[55–57] Also, with orientation of the axis and the tri-planar correction capacity of the closing wedge, plantarflexion or dorsiflexion can be "built in" to the osteotomy so as to further stabilize the forefoot upon correction.

The proximal chevron osteotomy without modification is purely translational. Subsequently correction capacity is based on the width of the proximal metatarsal shaft. Sammarco[36,58–60] modified the chevron by incorporating an opening wedge principle for his base procedure, therefore adding the rotational component to the correction. The large contact area allows for adequate screw or plate fixation or combination with k-wire. A level II investigation comparing the proximal chevron to the crescentic denoted adequate correction for both, but a significant difference in dorsiflexion malunion between the two with a 0% incidence for the chevron versus 17% incidence for the crescentic.[48]

OSTEOTOMY VERSUS ARTHRODESIS

The debate about whether or not to perform a Lapidus has to do with the biomechanical domain of hallux valgus. The individual ideology of each surgeon drives the choice of metatarsal base osteotomy versus fusion. However, depending on the case, Lapidus fusion and the proximal metatarsal osteotomy each has a role in hallux valgus correction. The key in this decision is to differentiate a case of a truly unstable first ray or medial column from a case of a hypermobile first ray secondary to development of hallux valgus. Determining this assertive differentiation is beyond the scope of this article. We will, however, review the biomechanical supporting arguments for the metatarsal basilar osteotomies, and assert that, at times, it is *this* chicken before *that* egg. In addition, it is the authors' belief, supported by a significant volume of evidence-based literature, that not every case of hallux valgus is hypermobile.

Morton,[61] in 1928, first introduced the theory of first-ray hypermobility. The causative connection between first-ray hypermobility and hallux valgus deformity was then asserted by Lapidus.[62,63] Contrary to widespread belief, neither investigator quantified hypermobility.[64] Klaue[65] designed an external caliper for the measurement of first-ray mobility, and this was later validated by Jones.[66] Klaue and Jones further defined the first ray as hypermobile if there were 9 mm or more of sagittal motion as measured with this device.

Others have shown an association between hallux valgus and an increased mobility of the first ray.[67–69] The numeric value or quantity of first-ray mobility had not been reported preoperatively or postoperatively in these studies, even amidst contention that a hypermobile first ray is indication enough for a first-metatarsal–cuneiform fusion.[64] In studies by Dreeben and Mann[70] and by Veri and colleagues,[71] DSTR and proximal first-metatarsal osteotomy for treatment of hallux valgus had low recurrence rates at both intermediate and long-term follow-up, indicating correction was maintained despite failure to fuse the first tarsometatarsal articulation.

In a recent cadaver study of specimens with hallux valgus deformity, a 50% reduction in sagittal plane mobility (to 5.2 mm from 11 mm) was observed following a distal soft tissue realignment DSTR and proximal first-metatarsal osteotomy.[72] Additionally, a recent prospective clinical study of 108 patients with hallux valgus and metatarsus primus varus was published.[64] Increased preoperative mobility of the first ray was regularly and consistently reduced to a normal range following proximal crescentic osteotomy and DSTR and without fusion of the first tarsometatarsal joint.[64] These studies further suggest that realignment of the first ray and reorientation of the soft tissue support structures, whether by soft tissue releases/transfers and osteotomies or by first-tarsometatarsal fusion is the crucial step in metatarsus primus varus and hallux valgus correction.

The corrective power of first-ray realignment and soft tissue balancing is demonstrated time and again in the rheumatoid foot reconstruction. Frequently, in addition to severe hallux valgus and lesser metatarsophalangeal joint dislocations, there is proximal first-tarsometatarsal instability demonstrated on radiograph (**Figs. 7** and **8**). Once the soft tissues are rebalanced and the first ray realigned, the proximal instability is reduced and stabilized (**Fig. 9**) without the need of proximal joint arthrodesis.

Another study by Kim and colleagues,[73] of 82 proximal chevron osteotomies and DSTR for symptomatic hallux valgus, showed clinical dorsiflexion mobility of the first ray to be reduced with clinical significance at an average of 1-year postoperative follow-up. They concluded that, secondary to stability of the first ray imparted by correction of the realignment metatarsal base osteotomy and DSTR, the surgical indication for the proximal osteotomy procedure can be recommended more broadly to include the correction of hallux valgus deformity accompanying first-ray hypermobility instead of the Lapidus procedure, which has more complications and a lower satisfaction rate.

These studies and many more suggest a stabilizing effect created by realignment of bone and soft tissue structures along the first-ray axis. There is a retrograde loading phenomenon that is reestablished back into the first tarsometatarsal joint, thus reducing the degree of preoperative "hypermobility." The stabilizing forces of the windlass mechanism of the plantar fascia, as well as the pull of the peroneus longus

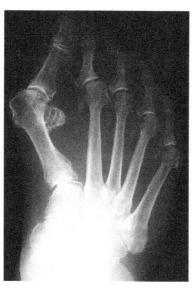

Fig. 7. Dorsal-plantar radiograph of weight-bearing right foot shows rheumatoid foot deformity with severe hallux valgus and proximal first-tarsometatarsal instability.

tendon at the first metatarsal base, are thought to be keys in first-ray stability without fusion.

Moving forward, one parameter proposed to assess sagittal plane instability at the first tarsometatarsal is the metatarsal-medial cuneiform angle or plantar gapping/wedging seen on the lateral weight-bearing foot radiograph.[74] It has not, however, been assessed in relationship to actual quantified mobility of the first ray.[64] In the

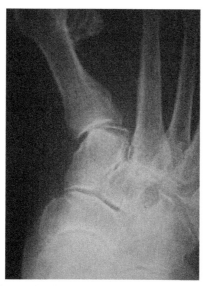

Fig. 8. Dorsal-plantar radiograph of weight-bearing right foot with focused view on first tarsometatarsal with joint incongruity.

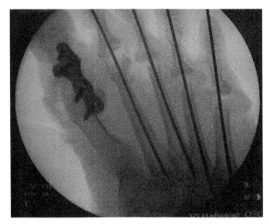

Fig. 9. Dorsal-plantar radiograph of simulated weight-bearing right foot. Intraoperative fluoroscopy view demonstrates proximal joint reduction via correction and balancing of distal deformities.

recent Coughlin and Jones study,[64] 23% of the feet demonstrated preoperative plantar gapping on radiograph (**Fig. 10**). Those with gapping had, on average, a significantly greater hallux valgus deformity than those without preoperative gapping. There was, however, no significant difference between those with and those without preoperative plantar gapping with respect to the mobility of the first ray. In the study group, the gapping resolved following realignment of the first ray in one third of the feet. There was no difference in the mean preoperative hallux valgus angle between the feet with residual gapping and those in which the gapping resolved. The group with residual gapping tended to have a larger angular correction compared with those in which gapping resolved. The mean mobility of the first ray was slightly higher both preoperatively and postoperatively in the group in which gapping resolved. Again, the findings of this study suggest a stabilizing effect is created by successfully realigning the first-ray axis by, in this case, proximal metatarsal osteotomy. These studies strongly suggest stability of the first ray can be achieved successfully and correction can be maintained when the imbalances of bone and soft tissue are corrected. This may be done with distal soft tissue rebalancing procedures combined with proximal metatarsal osteotomy and not necessarily a first-tarsometatarsal arthrodesis.

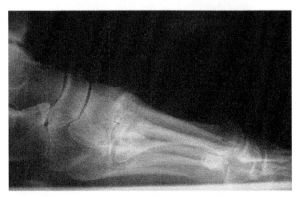

Fig. 10. Lateral radiograph of weight-bearing right foot. Mild plantar first tarsometatarsal joint gapping presumed suggestive of joint hypermobility or instability.

Meanwhile, many investigators have asserted that ankle equinus, as well as pes planus deformity, is also associated with the development of hallux valgus.[75–77] In more recent studies, no correlation was noted between limited preoperative ankle dorsiflexion and the magnitude of the preoperative or postoperative hallux valgus deformity, the magnitude of the angular correction, the postoperative AOFAS, or the postoperative subjective satisfaction of the patient.[64]

Sarrafian and others[68,78,79] have identified the plantar aponeurosis as a key component of first-ray stability. Coughlin[64] suggests that the realignment of the first ray restores the normal anatomic relationships and function of the intrinsic muscles, the extrinsic muscles, and the plantar aponeurosis, and that this leads to a reduction in first-ray mobility. It is thought that the stability of the first ray is a function of the alignment of the first ray and is not an intrinsic characteristic of the first metatarsocuneiform joint. This really is the crux in on-going discussions regarding the nature and appropriateness of the proximal first-metatarsal osteotomy in conjunction with DSTR for treatment of hallux valgus deformity.

In a recent forum, Drs. Donald Green and Peter Kim[80] eloquently describe their approach to hallux valgus. They state the obvious advantage to the metatarsal basilar osteotomy as allowing for continued natural range of motion throughout the rest of the joints in the foot. They further describe the foot's "tensegrity" as part of an integrated truss system where there are only tension and compression elements rather than levers or bending moments and without any torque at the joints.[81] This creates a mechanically efficient system that stores and returns energy with smooth motion in an efficient gait pattern with muscles developing tension on the fascia to provide protection, energy return, and smooth motion.[80] They further relate that arthrodesis leads to disintegration of gait with increased energy consumption, decreased gait speed, and increased pressure on other joints. They point to the example of ankle arthrodesis and its sequelae on adjacent joint health.

SUMMARY

These arguments and review of the literature are not meant to suggest the Lapidus arthrodesis has no role in hallux valgus correction or first-ray stabilization. This procedure can be used effectively and efficiently for both. This discussion is meant to simply point out that proximal osteotomies and soft tissue rebalancing can also successfully accomplish these goals. Each case of hallux valgus is different and has a unique etiology. A procedure should be selected only after this etiology is properly identified and evaluated.

The quest for definitive, irrefutable etiologic definition of the common hallux valgus foot deformity continues. To date, no all-encompassing theory or clinically proven entity has emerged to settle the debate in regards to pathologic first-ray hypermobility and its role in hallux valgus deformity and correction. We present a discussion on the use of proximal first-ray osteotomies in the surgical treatment for hallux valgus as a valid option compared with first-tarsometatarsal arthrodesis. Recent and historical literature tells us that stability of the first ray is a function of the alignment and reestablishment of retrograde stabilizing forces at the first tarsometatarsal joint. This realignment and stabilization may be accomplished with the use of distal soft tissue and proximal osteotomy procedures.

REFERENCES

1. Sim Fook L, Hodgson AR. A comparison of foot forms among the non-shoe and shoe-wearing Chinese population. J Bone Joint Surg Am 1958;40-A:1058–62.

2. Coughlin MJ, Thompson FM. The high price of high fashion footwear. Instr Course Lect 1995;44:371–7.
3. Reverdin J. De la deviation en dehors du gros orl (hallux valgus) et son traitement chirurgical. Trans Int Med Congress 1881;2:408–12 [in French].
4. Mayo CH. The surgical treatment of bunion. Ann Surg 1908;48:300–2.
5. Keller WL. The surgical treatment of bunions and hallux valgus. NY Med 1904;80: 741–2.
6. Brandes M. Zur operation therapie des hallux valgus. [For the surgical therapy of hallux valgus]. Zentralbl Chir 1924;56:243–4 [in German].
7. Austin DW, Leventen EO. A new osteotomy for hallux valgus. Clin Orthop 1981; 157:25–30.
8. Corless JR. A modification of the Mitchell procedure. J Bone Joint Surg 1976;58-B: 128–32.
9. Johnson KA, Cofield RH, Morrey BF. Chevron osteotomy for hallux valgus. Clin Orthop 1979;142:44–7.
10. Mann RA, Coughlin MJ. Adult hallux valgus. In: Coughlin MJ, Mann RA, editors. Surgery of the foot and ankle. 7th edition. St. Louis (MO): Mosby; 1999. p. 150–269.
11. Myerson MS. Hallux valgus. In: Meyerson MS, editor. Foot and ankle disorders. Philadelphia: Saunders; 2000. p. 213–88.
12. Richardson EG, Donley BG. Disorders of hallux. In: Canle ST, editor. Campbell's operative orthopaedics. 10th edition. Philadelphia: Mosby; 2003. p. 3915–4015.
13. Badwey TM, Dutkowsky JP, Graves SC, et al. An anatomical basis for the degree of displacement of the distal chevron osteotomy in the treatment of hallux valgus. Foot Ankle Int 1997;18:213–5.
14. Harper MC. Correction of metatarsus primus varus with the chevron metatarsal osteotomy. Clin Orthop 1989;243:180–3.
15. Jahss MH, Troy AI, Kummer F. Roentgenographic and mathematical analysis of first metatarsal osteotomies for metatarsus primus varus: a comparative study. Foot Ankle Int 1985;5:280–321.
16. Sarrafian SK. A method of predicting the degree of functional correction of the metatarsus primus varus with a distal lateral displacement osteotomy in hallux valgus. Foot Ankle Int 1985;5:322–6.
17. Miller S, Croce WA. The Austin procedure for surgical correction of hallux abducto valgus deformity. J Am Podiatry Assoc 1979;69:110–8.
18. Hattrup SJ, Johnson KA. Chevron osteotomy: analysis of factors in patients' dissatisfaction. Foot Ankle 1985;5:327–32.
19. Muhlbauer M, Zembsch A, Trnka HJ. Kurzfristige ergebnisse der modifizierten chevron-osteotomie mit weichteiltechnik und bohrdrahtfixation—eine prospective studie. [Short-term results of modified chevron osteotomy with soft tissue technique and guide wire fixation—a prospective study]. Z Orthop Ihre Grenzgeb 2001;139:435–9 [in German].
20. Weil LS. Scarf osteotomy for correction of hallux valgus. Historical perspective, surgical technique, and results. Foot Ankle Clin 2000;5:559–80.
21. Zygmont KHZ, Gudas CJ, Laros GS. Bunionectomy with intertarsal screw fixation. J Am Podiatr Med Assoc 1989;79:322–9.
22. Barouk LS. Scarf oteotomy for hallux valgus correction. Local anatomy, surgical technique, and combination with other forefoot procedures. Foot Ankle Clin 2000;5(3):525–58.
23. Pollack RA, Bellacosa RA, Higgins KR, et al. Critical evaluation of the short "Z" bunionectomy. J Foot Surg 1989;28:158–61.
24. Barouk LS. Osteotomies of the great toe. J Foot Surg 1992;31:388–99.

25. Kristen KH, Berger C, Stelzig S, et al. The SCARF osteotomy for the correction of hallux valgus deformities. Foot Ankle Int 2002;23:221–9.

26. Coetzee JC. Scarf osteotomy for hallux valgus correction: the dark side. Foot Ankle Int 2003;24:29–33.

27. Trnka, HJ. Osteotomies for hallux valgus correction. 10:15–33, 2005.

28. Coetzee JC, Rippstein P. Surgical strategies: scarf osteotomy for hallux valgus. Foot Ankle Int 2007;28(4):529–35.

29. Deenik AR, Pilot P, Brandt SE, et al. Scarf versus chevron osteotomy in hallux valgus: a randomized controlled trial in 96 patients. Foot Ankle Int 2007;28(5): 537–41.

30. Hyer CF, Glover JP, Berlet GC, et al. A comparison of the crescentic and Mau osteotomies for correction of hallux valgus. J Foot Ankle Surg 2008;47(2): 103–11.

31. Pehlivan O, Akmaz I, Solakoglu C, et al. Proximal oblique crescentic osteotomy in hallux valgus. J Am Podiatr Med Assoc 2004;94(1):43–6.

32. Loison M. Note sure letraitment chirurgical du hallux valgus d'apres l'etude radiographique de la deformation. Bul Soc Chir Paris 1901;27:528–31 [in French].

33. Balacescu J. Un caz de hallux valgus simetric. Rev Chir 1903;7:128–35.

34. Trethowan J. Hallux valgus. In: Choyce CC, editor. A system of surgery. New York: Hoeber, PG; 1923. p. 1046–9.

35. McClusky LC, Johnson JE, Wynarsky GT, et al. Comparison of stability of proximal crescentic metatarsal osteotomy and proximal horizontal "V" osteotomy. Foot Ankle Int 1994;15(5):263–70.

36. Easley ME, Kiebzak GM, Davis WH, et al. Prospective, randomized comparison of proximal crescentic and proximal chevron osteotomies for correction of hallux valgus deformity. Foot Ankle Int 1996;17(6):307–16.

37. Markbreiter LA, Thompson FM. Proximal metatarsal osteotomy in hallux valgus correction: a comparison of crescentic and chevron procedures. Foot Ankle Int 1997;18(2):71–6.

38. Vora AM, Myerson MS. First metatarsal osteotomy nonunion and malunion. Foot Ankle Clin 2005;10(1):35–54.

39. Chiodo CP, Schon LC, Myerson MS. Clinical results with the Ludloff osteotomy for correction of adult hallux valgus. Foot Ankle Int 2004;25(8):532–6.

40. Saxena A, McCammon D. The Ludloff osteotomy: a critical analysis. J Foot Ankle Surg 1997;36(2):100–5.

41. Mann RA, Rudicel S, Graves SC. Repair of hallux valgus with a distal soft-tissue procedure and proximal metatarsal osteotomy. A long-term follow-up. J Bone Joint Surg Am 1992;74(1):124–9.

42. Thorardson DB, Leventen EO. Hallux valgus correction with proximal metatarsal osteotomy: two-year follow-up. Foot Ankle 1992;13(6):321–6.

43. Bar-David T, Greenburg PM. Retrospective analysis of the Mau osteotomy and effect of a fibular sesamoidectomy. J Foot Ankle Surg 1998;37(3):212–6.

44. Neese DJ, Zelichowski JE, Patton GW. Mau osteotomy: an alternative procedure to the closing abductory base wedge osteotomy. J Foot Surg 1982;28(4):352–62.

45. Deorio JK, Ware AW. Single absorbable polydioxanone pin fixation for distal chevron bunion osteotomies. Foot Ankle Int 2001;22:832–5.

46. Zettl R, Trnka HJ, Easley M, et al. Moderate to severe hallux valgus deformity: correction with proximal crescentic osteotomy and distal soft-tissue release. Arch Orthop Trauma Surg 2000;120:397–402.

47. Lian GJ, Markolf K, Cracchiolo A. Strength of fixation constructs for basilar osteotomies of the first metatarsal. Foot Ankle 1992;13:509.

48. Jones C, Coughlin M, Villadot R, et al. Proximal crescentic metatarsal osteotomy: the effect of saw blade orientation on first ray elevation. Foot Ankle Int 2005;26: 152–7.

49. Cohen M, Roman A, Ayres M, et al. The crescentic shelf osteotomy. J Foot Ankle Surg 1993;33:204–26.

50. Gallentine JW, DeOrio JK, DeOrio MJ. Bunion surgery using locking-plate fixation of proximal metatarsal chevron osteotomies. Foot Ankle Int 2007;28(3):361–8.

51. Trnka HJ, Parks BG, Ivanic G, et al. Six first metatarsal shaft osteotomies: mechanical and immobilization comparisons. Clin Orthop Relat Res 2000;381: 256–65.

52. Acevedo JI, Sammarco VJ, Boucher HR, et al. Mechanical comparison of cyclic loading in five different first metatarsal shaft osteotomies. Foot Ankle Int 2002; 23(8):711–6.

53. Ludloff K. Die beseitigung des hallux valgus durch die schraege planta-dorsale osteotomie des metatarsus. I Arch Klin Chir 1918;110:364–87 [in German].

54. Trnka HJ, Hofstaetter SG, Hofstaetter JG, et al. Intermediate-term results of the Ludloff osteotomy in one hundred and eleven feet. J Bone Joint Surg Am 2008; 90:531–9.

55. Resch S, Stenstrom A, Egund N. Proximal closing wedge osteotomy and adductor tenotomy for treatment of hallux valgus. Foot Ankle 1989;9:272–80.

56. Trnka HJ, Muhlbauer M, Zembsch A, et al. Basal closing wedge osteotomy for correction of hallux valgus and metatarsus primus varus: 10–22 year follow-up. Foot Ankle Int 1999;20:171–7.

57. Zembsch A, Trnka HJ, Ritschl P. Correction of hallux valgus. Metatarsal osteotomy versus excision arthroplasty. Clin Orthop 2000;376:183–94.

58. Sammarco GJ, Brainard BJ, Sammarco VJ. Bunion correction using proximal chevron osteotomy. Foot Ankle 1993;14:8–14.

59. Sammarco GJ, Conti SF. Proximal chevron metatarsal osteotomy: single incision technique. Foot Ankle 1993;14:44–7.

60. Sammarco GJ, Russo-Alexi FG. Bunion correction using proximal chevron osteotomy: a single incision technique. Foot Ankle Int 1998;19:430–7.

61. Morton DJ. Hypermobility of the first metatarsal bone: the interlinking factor between metatarsalgia and longitudinal arch strains. J Bone Joint Surg 1928; 10:187–96.

62. Lapidus PW. A quarter of a century of experience with the operative correction of the metatarsus varus primus in hallux valgus. Bull Hosp Joint Dis 1956;17: 404–21.

63. Lapidus PW. The author's bunion operation from 1931–1959. Clin Orthop Relat Res 1960;16:119–35.

64. Coughlin MJ, Jones CP. Hallux valgus and first ray mobility, a prospective study. J Bone Joint Surg Am 2007;89-A(9):1887–98.

65. Klaue K, Hansen ST, Masquelet AC. Clinical, quantitative assessment of first tarsometatarsal mobility in the sagittal plane and its relation to hallux valgus deformity. Foot Ankle Int 1994;15:9–13.

66. Jones CP, Coughlin MJ, Pierce-Villadot R, et al. The validity and reliability of the Klaue device. Foot Ankle Int 2005;26:951–6.

67. Glasoe WM, Allen MK, Saltzman CL. First ray dorsal mobility in relation to hallux valgus deformity and first intermetatarsal angle. Foot Ankle Int 2001;22:98–101.

68. Grebing BR, Coughlin MJ. The effect of ankle position on the exam for first ray mobility. Foot Ankle Int 2004;25:467–75.

69. Grebing BR, Coughlin MJ. Evaluation of Morton's theory of second metatarsal hypertrophy. J Bone Joint Surg Am 2004;86:1375–86.
70. Dreeben S, Mann RA. Advanced hallux valgus deformity: long-term results utilizing the distal soft tissue procedure and proximal metatarsal osteotomy. Foot Ankle Int 1996;17:142–4.
71. Veri JP, Pirani SP, Claridge R. Crescentic proximal metatarsal osteotomy for moderate to severe hallux valgus: a mean 12.2 year follow-up study. Foot Ankle Int 2001;22:817–22.
72. Coughlin MJ, Jones CP, Viladot R, et al. Hallux valgus and first ray mobility: a cadaveric study. Foot Ankle Int 2004;25:537–44.
73. Kim JY, Park JS, Hwang SK, et al. Mobility changes of the first ray after hallux valgus surgery: clinical results after proximal metatarsal chevron osteotomy and distal soft tissue procedure. Foot Ankle Int 2008;29:468–72.
74. King DM, Toolan BC. Associated deformities and hypermobility in hallux valgus: an investigation with weightbearing radiographs. Foot Ankle Int 2004;25:251–5.
75. Morton DJ. The human foot; its evolution, physiology and functional disorders. New York: Columbia University Press; 1935.
76. Hansen ST Jr. Hallux valgus surgery. Morton and Lapidus were right! Clin Podiatr Med Surg 1996;13:347–54.
77. Hansen ST Jr. Functional reconstruction of the foot and ankle. Philadelphia: Lippincott Williams and Wilkins; 2000. p. 221.
78. Sarrafian SK. Functional characteristics of the foot and plantar aponeurosis under tibiotalar loading. Foot Ankle 1987;8:4–18.
79. Rush SM, Christensen JC, Johnson CH. Biomechanics of the first ray. Part II: metatarsus primus varus as a cause of hypermobility. A three-dimensional kinematic analysis in a cadaver model. J Foot Ankle Surg 2000;39:68–77.
80. Green DR, Kim P. Should the Lapidus replace the closing base wedge osteotomy? Podiatry Today. Malvem: HMP Communications LLC; 2004. p. 56–60.
81. Levin S. On your toes—tensegrity for terpsichore. Foot Biomechanics and Orthotic Therapy. Dec 1–3, Las Vegas (NV).

The Versatility of the Lapidus Arthrodesis

Neal M. Blitz, DPM, FACFAS

KEYWORDS

- Lapidus arthrodesis • Midfoot fusion
- Morton's foot • Hallux valgus • Bunionectomy

Lapidus arthrodesis is probably the most versatile procedure of the foot and ankle surgeon. Although the procedure was conceived initially for the surgical treatment of met primus adductus associated with hallux valgus, it has also been used for the treatment of a variety of other conditions.[1–6] These conditions include hallux limitus, revision bunion surgery, medial column stabilization, and other conditions shown in **Box 1**. A complete understanding the Lapidus' advantages, disadvantages, and its limitations is necessary for successful implementation of the Lapidus approach.

THE LAPIDUS IN METATARSUS PRIMUS ADDUCTUS WITH HALLUX VALGUS

The Lapidus procedure, mainstreamed by Dr. Paul Lapidus, is best known for its use with primary metatarsal primus adductus with hallux valgus.[4–6] The procedure may involve an isolated fusion of the first tarsometatarsal (TMT) joint (**Fig. 1**) or incorporate the second metatarsal base into the fusion (**Fig. 2**). Although Dr. Lapidus initially described a concomitant fusion of the second metatarsal base, most surgeons do not typically include this additional fusion. In some situations, the second metatarsal base or intermediate cuneiform may be temporarily spanned with fixation to add more stability during the healing process (**Fig. 3**). The procedure/technique and fixation construct has evolved significantly since its inception, but most advances have been gained since Sangeorzan and Hansen reported on two-crossed screw fixation of the fusion site in 1989.[7]

The benefit of performing a Lapidus for hallux valgus is that the procedure addresses the problem at the apex of the deformity, increases the efficiency of Peroneus Longus, and stabilizes the medial column.[8,9] There are several technical aspects of the procedure that are important to review that may improve outcomes (**Fig. 4**).

LAPIDUS TECHNICAL PEARLS (SCREW FIXATION)

The fusion site is accessed through a dorsomedial curvilinear incision, and the medial dorsal cutaneous nerve is avoided. Access to the first TMT may be achieved with

Department of Orthopaedic Surgery, Bronx-Lebanon Hospital Center, 1650 Selwyn Avenue, Bronx, NY 10457, USA
E-mail address: nealblitz@yahoo.com

Clin Podiatr Med Surg 26 (2009) 427–441
doi:10.1016/j.cpm.2009.03.009
0891-8422/09/$ – see front matter © 2009 Elsevier Inc. All rights reserved.

> **Box 1**
> **Conditions where lapidus has been implemented**
>
> Primary met primus adductus with hallux valgus
>
> Revision hallux valgus surgery
>
> Hallux limitus
>
> Forefoot overload (hypermobility syndrome)
>
> Morton's foot reconstruction
>
> Medial column stabilization with pes planus
>
> Distracting procedure for short first ray
>
> Arthrosis of the first TMT joint
>
> Primary fusion for comminuted first TMT fracture

a linear or transverse capsulotomy (see **Fig. 4**A), avoiding the ligament that extends to the second metatarsal base if an isolated first TMT fusion is being performed. Resection of the first TMT with osteotomes and curettes avoids thermal necrosis of bone (see **Fig. 4**B) that may occur with saw resection. Also, the subchondral plate is preserved to provide stability to the fixation and is perforated with a bone pic to allow boney ingress necessary for fusion to occur[10] (see **Fig. 4**C). It is important to either translate or plantarflex the first metatarsal on the medial cuneiform to accommodate for the shortening inherent with the joint resection. The intermetatarsal angle is reduced manually. This particular fixation construct calls for at least two screws to be placed across the arthrodesis site (see **Fig. 4**D and E). The distal-to-proximal screw is placed first with lag technique originating on the dorsal aspect of the first metatarsal, oriented so that the screw's long axis is nearly perpendicular to the fusion site (theoretically increasing the compressive force of the screw). The second screw, originating on the dorsal aspect of the medial cuneiform, may or may not be placed with lag technique. A locally derived stress-relieving bone graft may assist with healing of the fusion (see **Fig. 4**F).

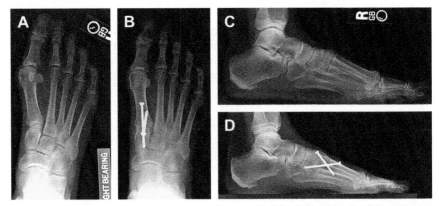

Fig. 1. Isolated first TMT joint fusion (modified Lapidus bunionectomy)—the two-crossed screw technique. (*A, C*) Preoperative weightbearing radiographs. (*B, D*) Postoperative weightbearing radiographs. Two long 3.5-mm fully threaded cortical screws are used to maintain the fusion site.

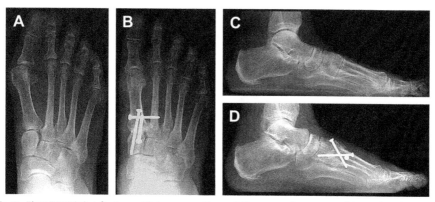

Fig. 2. First TMT joint fusion with incorporation of the second metatarsal base. (*A, C*) Preoperative weightbearing radiographs. (*B, D*) Postoperative weightbearing radiographs. When this concomitant fusion is desired, debridement of the medial second metatarsal base is necessary for fusion. A screw is placed permanently from the first metatarsal base into to the second metatarsal base to stabilize the fusion.

The ability of the Lapidus arthrodesis to achieve intermetatarsal angle correction is well documented throughout the literature.[11–18] In a critical retrospective evaluation of the modified Lapidus procedure, McInnes and Bouche reported that a postoperative intermetatarsal angle of 10° or less resulted in a satisfactory/good clinical outcome.[11] In addition to intermetatarsal angle correction, the Lapidus arthrodesis may be combined with other first-ray procedures to correct for multilevel first ray deformities, such as proximal intra-articular set angle or hallux interphalangeus (**Fig. 5**). In recent years, more studies are emerging that examine the surgeon experience, pain reduction, and patient satisfaction after a Lapidus arthrodesis.

A retrospective study evaluating the Lapidus in 32 patients by Kopp and colleagues[16] in 2005 found a 93% satisfactory rate in terms of pain improvement, 86% were satisfied with the cosmetic appearance, and 83% would repeat the

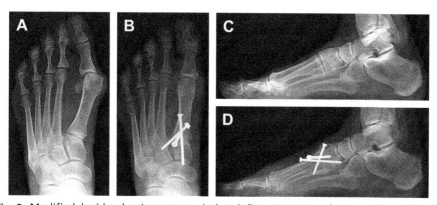

Fig. 3. Modified lapidus bunionectomy—isolated first TMT joint fusion with additional "temporary" screw into the intermediate cuneiform. (*A, C*) Preoperative weightbearing radiographs. (*B, D*) Postoperative weightbearing radiographs. Placing an additional screw into the intermediate cuneiform stabilizes the construct. This screw typically is removed once isolated fusion of the first TMT joint is achieved.

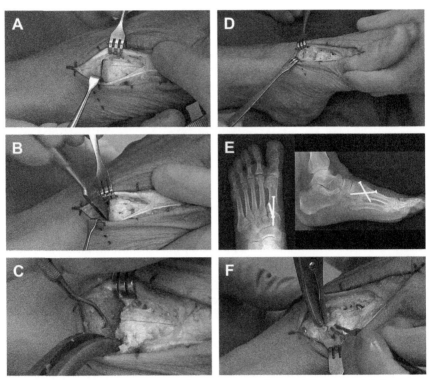

Fig. 4. Surgical technique for isolated first TMT joint fusion. (*A*) First TMT joint exposed through a longitudinal capsulotomy. (*B*) Osteotomes/curettage joint resection keeping the subchondral plate intact. (*C*) Subchondral plate perforation. Bone pic is used to avoid thermal necrosis. (*D*) Fixated first TMT fusion. (*E*) Radiographs show two crossed screw technique. (*F*) Local stress-relieving bone graft placed at the joint line.

procedure. The technique involved two screws and a non-weightbearing protocol. The mean intermetatarsal angle improved from 16° preoperatively to 6° postoperatively. Statistical significance (*P*<.001) was achieved in both the average visual analog pain score (preoperative 7.2, postoperative 2.3) and the American Orthopaedic Foot and Ankle Society Hallux Metatarsophalangeal Interphalangeal Score (preoperative 44.8, postoperative 87.3). Complications included one recurrent hallux valgus, two with symptomatic hallux varus, one deep vein thrombosis, and one fixation failure. Union rate was 100%.

In 2004, Rink-Brüne performed a respective review of the authors' first consecutive 106 patients with symptomatic hallux valgus (and mainly hypermobility).[17] Fixation involved a single 3.5-mm cannulated screw and a threaded Kirschner wire. Patients were nonweightbearing for 6 weeks postoperatively without the use of a cast. Union rate was 98.2%, and the mean postoperative intermetatarsal angle reduction was 12.4° with radiographic undercorrection in 4.7% of patients. Overall complication rate was 5.7%. Nearly three quarters of the patients completed a survey revealing that 70.5% were satisfied, and 80.2% would choose a Lapidus correction again.

A prospective outcome study performed by Coetzee and Wickum in 2004 evaluated the functional outcome of patients undergoing a Lapidus with moderate to severe hallux valgus (intermetatarsal angle >14°) in 105 feet (91 patients).[18] The American

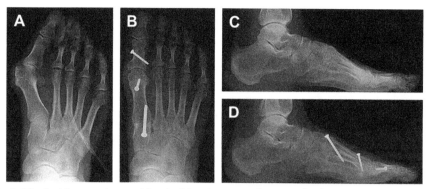

Fig. 5. The lapidus may be combined with other procedures on the first ray to correct structural deformities. (*A, C*) Preoperative weightbearing radiographs. (*B, D*) Postoperative weightbearing radiographs. The first ray is realigned—the Lapidus for intermetatarsal angle correction, the reverdin for proximal articular set angle correction, and the akin osteototomy for hallux interphalangeus correction. In this case, one of the Lapidus screws was removed after fusion was achieved.

Orthopaedic Foot and Ankle Society Hallux Metatarsophalangeal Interphalangeal Score improved from 52 preoperative to 87 postoperative, reaching statistical significance (*P*<.001). Mean intermetatarsal angle improved from 18° preoperative to 8.2° postoperative. Nonunion occurred in seven patients and loss of correction in five patients. A particularly interesting finding of this study is that a 0.3° increase in the intermetatarsal angle was identified between the 1 year and the mean 3.7 year follow-up. This suggests that a Lapidus may have the ability to maintain intermetatarsal angle correction in the short term, although long-term studies will be well received.

Popelka and colleagues[19,20] recently (2008) reported on their experience with the Lapidus in two separate publications. One review included 61 patients over a 4 year period undergoing a variety of fixation constructs (screws, Kirschner wires, or memory staples).[19] Seventy-three percent of patients reported no pain in the forefoot, 13% experienced pain in the "transverse arch," and one patient had a psuedoarthrosis. The American Orthopaedic Foot and Ankle Society score improved from 48.1 preoperatively to 89.2 postoperatively.

THE LAPIDUS WITH HALLUX LIMITUS

The surgical treatment of hallux limitus has mainly centered on distal osteotomies of the first metatarsal head to decompress the first metatarsophalangeal joint, and a fair number of studies involve such. Some surgeons advocate the use of the Lapidus for the treatment of hallux limitus, and it is theorized to be effective by decompressing the joint in a similar fashion to that of distal osteotomies, except at a more proximal location and performed through the fusion site.[21,22] It should be remembered that the first metatarsal is translated inferiorly or plantarflexed through the fusion site to compensate for the shortening with the procedure. Procedures at the first metatarsophalangeal joint may also be combined with a Lapidus, such as cheilectomy (exostectomy) or osteochondral lesion repair (**Fig. 6**). However, no studies specifically support the use of the Lapidus for hallux limitus and are the next logical steps.

However, with advancing arthrosis of the big toe joint, surgeons may not want to perform a Lapidus for hallux limitus in the event the procedure is ineffective, and a joint

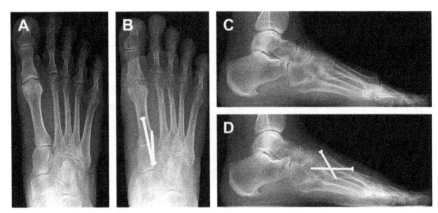

Fig. 6. The lapidus for hallux limitus. (*A, C*) Preoperative weightbearing radiographs. (*B, D*) Postoperative weightbearing radiographs. The Lapidus may be combined with cheilectomy. In this case, note how the elevation of the first ray is corrected postoperatively. (*Courtesy of* Dan Choung, DPM, San Rafael, California.)

destructive procedure at the first metatarsophalangeal joint may be needed. Studies and case reports in this area are also lacking. Fusion of the first metatarsophalangeal joint is preferred (by this author) over implant or Keller if a Lapidus precedes the non-salvageble arthrosis of the great toe joint.

THE LAPIDUS AND HYPERMOBILITY

Although the Lapidus procedure has been an indication to treat hypermobility with hallux valgus, the significance and surgical treatment of medial column hypermobility still remains an area of controversy.[23–27] Hypermobility has been associated with pes planus, metatarsus primus adductus, hallux valgus, midfoot arthrosis, metatarsalgia, and lesser metatarsal stress fractures.[23,28] Although most surgeons associate hypermobility with excessive sagittal plane excursion of the medial column, hypermobility (or instability) in the transverse plane may occur concomitantly as well. Based on two separate cadaveric studies, it appears that the first TMT is responsible for 41% to 57% of total medial column motion.[29,30] When the hypermobility is believed to be pathologic by the surgeon, the aforementioned cadaveric findings suggest that nearly half (give or take a little) of motion of the first ray will be reduced with an isolated fusion of the first TMT.

Although the Lapidus has been associated with treatment of hypermobility, it should be understood that metatarsal osteotomies are similarly as effective in managing the condition. A prospective, randomized study in 101 feet by Faber and colleagues[31] showed similar outcomes when a distal first metatarsal osteotomy (Hohmann type) was compared with the Lapidus procedure in patients with hypermobility. Coughlin and Jones noted that the hypermobility resolved after a cresentric osteotomy and distal soft tissue release in all but 2 of 23 patients as part of a prospective study.[32] In two separate cadaveric studies, reduction of the intermetatarsal angle by a distal metatarsal osteotomy or base osteotomy of the first metatarsal reduces first ray motion, and restoration of the windlass mechanism has been suggested as the mechanism for this finding.[33,34] Therefore, it appears to be critical to obtain reduction of the intermetatarsal angle regardless of the method of hallux valgus correction. The decision to treat the hypermobility through selective fusions depends on the following: degree of deformity (intermetatarsal angle), overall sagittal mobility, first ray position, ability to restore the windlass mechanism, transverse plane instability, first ray length, stigma of first ray insufficiency, and surgeon experience.[35]

When using the Lapidus for the management of hypermobility, it is beneficial to be aware of the "intraoperative hypermobility test."[35,36] The author described this intraoperative maneuver in 2005 to evaluate the transverse plane intermetatarsal angle reduction and sagittal plane reduction of first ray mobility when performing a Lapidus. (**Fig. 7**) In some instances, this test will guide the surgeon as to whether additional concomitant fusions should be considered.

LAPIDUS AS MEDIAL COLUMN STABILIZING PROCEDURE

Although the ability of the Lapidus to improve transverse plane deformity is well documented, there is a paucity of literature supporting the ability of the Lapidus to radiographically improve the sagittal plane alignment of the foot.[9] Recently, Avino and colleagues[9] showed that isolated first TMT fusion led to statistically significant ($P < .0001$) improvements of the talo–first metatarsal angle and medial cuneiform height in a retrospective radiographic review study of 39 feet. Although it is interesting that the angle the first metatarsal made with the floor in the sagittal plane (lateral metatarsal floor angle) did not have a significant change after Lapidus. Therefore, the investigators suggested that the improvement in the talo–first metatarsal angle (of approximately 3°) is the result of dorsiflexion of the talus and further correlated this occurrence with a previous cadaveric study illustrating this talar dorsiflexion after Lapidus.[8,9] Perhaps the locking mechanism of the first ray may play a role.[37] Talar dorsiflexion after Lapidus can be witnessed in clinical practice, as the talus will dorsally peak on the navicular on weightbearing radiographs (**Fig. 8**).

ROLE OF THE LAPIDUS IN MORTON'S FOOT RECONSTRUCTION AND FLAT FOOT RECONSTRUCTION

The concept of the Morton's foot was introduced by Dudley Morton, an anatomist. The features of the so-called Morton's foot include a short first metatarsal, hypermobility,

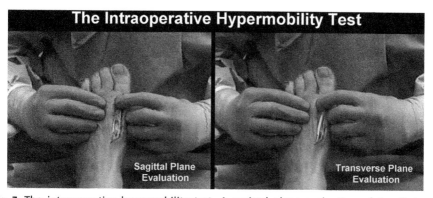

Fig. 7. The intraoperative hypermobility test. A sagittal plane evaluation of the first ray motion should be performed after the fixation is in place to ensure reduction of medial column mobility. Similarly, the transverse plane may be evaluated by placing the surgeon's index finger between the heads of the first and second metatarsals to ensure these segments do not overtly gap apart.

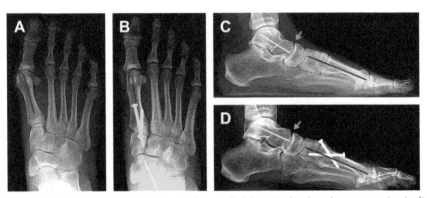

Fig. 8. The influence of the lapidus on the medial longitudinal arch. Improved talo-first metatarsal angle (*yellow and blue lines*) improvement is evident in this case. Here, the talus is propped up with stabilization of the arch (*orange arrows*). (*A, C*) Preoperative weight-bearing radiographs. (*B, D*) Postoperative weightbearing radiographs.

and equinus.[38–40] The nature of the Lapidus to stabilize (or treat) the pathologic hyper-mobility of the medial column has enabled the Lapidus arthrodesis to be a primary crucial competent of a "Morton's foot reconstruction." Although there is no standard procedure for a Morton's foot reconstruction, the concept is to balance the foot so that the medial column is stabilized and the parabola is restored, enabling the first meta-tarsal to reassume its role as a major weightbearing structure in the foot. Surgically, this typically takes the form of a Lapidus arthrodesis combined with lesser metatarsal shortening procedures along with digital corrections. (**Fig. 9**) Rearfoot realignment procedures may also be indicated as part of flat foot reconstruction (ie, posterior tibia-lis tendon dysfunction).[28,41–45]

THE DISTRACTION LAPIDUS

Lengthening the first ray through the first TMT joint has been advocated for surgically correcting the short first ray, often associated with the Morton's foot or failed

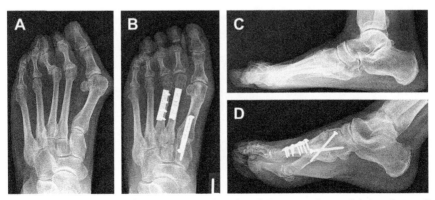

Fig. 9. Lapidus in Morton's foot reconstruction. (*A, C*) Preoperative weightbearing radiographs show short first ray with long second and third metatarsals with dorsally dislocated associated digits. Hallux abductovalgus present. (*B, D*) Postoperative radiographs after Lap-idus arthrodesis combined with diaphyseal shortening osteotomies to restore the parabola and stabilize the medial column. (*Courtesy of* Dan Choung, DPM, San Rafael, California).

bunionectomies in which the first ray has been previously shortened.[28] The procedure involves incorporating an intercalary bone graft into the first TMT fusion site to lengthen the segment (**Fig. 10**). The length of bone graft varies and depends on the clinical scenario. The graft size ranges from 0.5 cm to 1.5 cm, with 1.0 cm probably being the most likely graft size to be used. The surgeon, however, will balance the amount of distraction against the overall parabola length. It is possible to distract the segment to cause jamming of the big toe joint, so surgeons should be cognizant of this potential occurrence and monitor the first metatarsophalangeal joint range of motion intraoperatively. Acute distraction greater than 2 cm could potentially result in neurovascular compromise.

The concept of distraction of the first ray is not a new concept, and other methods of achieving this distraction have included the scarf metatarsal osteotomy and callus distraction.[46–48] Although clinical studies are lacking and the literature is limited, it mainly consists of retrospective reviews of a small number of patients. Hamilton and colleagues[49] performed a multicenter study of 17 feet that underwent a bone-block distraction for symptomatic Lapidus nonunion. All but one patient had autogenous ipsilateral bone-block graft harvested from either the calcaneus or the distal tibia. Fixation involved screws, or combination of screws and a dorsal or dorsomedial plate. There was no mention of the bone-block graft length. Of this revisional surgery patient population that included seven smokers out of the 17 feet, a overall successful fusion was achieved in 82% of feet (14 feet) after a minimum of 6 months.

THE LAPIDUS IN REVISION BUNION SURGERY

The Lapidus procedure has been used also as a salvage operation for correcting failed (or recurrent) hallux valgus surgery initially treated with a distal or proximal first metatarsal osteotomy. Although there are many reasons for a failure of a metatarsal osteotomy procedure, it is the Lapidus procedure that may be best suited for realigning the first ray. If there was untreated hypermobility at the first TMT joint, then the Lapidus should address some or most of that residual instability.[35] In some cases, it may be

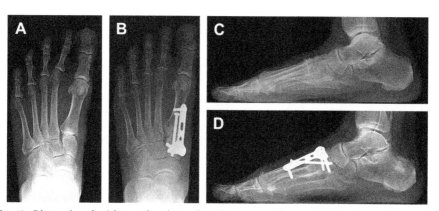

Fig. 10. Distraction lapidus arthrodesis. (*A, C*) Preoperative weightbearing radiographs. Arthritic first TMT joint with long second metatarsal. (*B, D*) Postoperative healed weight-bearing radiographs. An arthritic joint often requires a greater joint resection to reach bleeding subchondral bone; therefore, a short first ray will be that much shorter if not addressed. A dorsal medial plate secures the harvested ipsilateral autogenous calcaneal bone block. Note the restoration of the parabola with the distraction Lapidus (without second metatarsal shortening).

advantageous to perform the revision bunion surgery at the first TMT joint (instead of at the previous metatarsal osteotomy site), especially if the index surgery site is devitalized. Most iatrogenic positional deformities can be corrected through a Lapidus arthrodesis.

In 2003, Coetzee published results on a prospective functional outcome and patient satisfaction study of the Lapidus procedure for the correction of symptomatic failed hallux valgus in 24 patients (26 feet).[50] The residual transverse plane deformity correction was achieved through the Lapidus fusion (mean intermetatarsal angle, preoperatively 18° to postoperatively 8.6°). From the patient standpoint, approximately three quarters of the patients were very satisfied, and there were no dissatisfied patients. This study provides evidence that the Lapidus arthrodesis may be an effective method of treatment of the failed bunionectomy.

When considering the "failed Bunionectomy", however, it should be understood that the first metatarsal may have attained iatrogenic intrinsic structural deformity from the index operation. Although the Lapidus may be used in many situations regarding the failed bunionectomy, there are several modifications to the procedure/technique of which the surgeon should be aware.

Sagittal plane deformities are most often seen after base wedge osteotomies that undergo plastic deformation from premature postoperative weightbearing, or a poorly executed transverse base wedge with wire fixation. The elevated first ray may result in functional hallux limitus as well as incite the stigmata of first ray insufficiency (hammer toes, lesser metatarsal overload). If the apex of the intrinsic deformity of the first metatarsal is near the base (ie, close to the first TMT joint) then the fulcrum for the angulation is potentially greater and may be more difficult to correct. The surgeon compensates for this by performing a translatory (with or without plantarflexory) Lapidus fusion. Of course there is a limit with which one can translate the first metatarsal on the medial cuneiform and still maintain enough bone-to-bone contact and stabilization to attain a proper fusion. In my experience, the amount of translation that can be successfully achieved is approximately 50% of the joint. Depending on the clinical scenario, it may be necessary to perform ancillary procedures to balance the foot (**Fig. 11**).

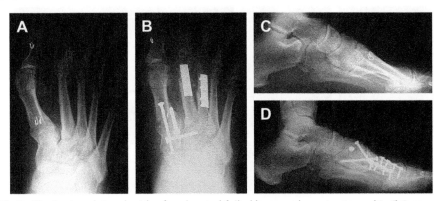

Fig. 11. Plantar translatory lapidus for elevated failed base wedge osteotomy. (*A, C*) Preoperative weightbearing radiographs. Previous transverse base wedge osteotomy with monofilament wire resulted in elevated first ray and recurrent bunion. First ray is short in comparison with lesser metatarsals. (*B, D*) Postoperative weightbearing radiographs. After a plantar translatory lapidus (approximately 40% in this case), the center of the first met head is in line with the bisection of the talus on the lateral view. Concomitant diaphyseal shortening osteotomies were performed to restore the parabola.

PRIMARY FUSION FOR TARSOMETATARSAL FRACTURE

It is generally agreed that intra-articular fractures lead to traumatic arthrosis, with more severe fractures more likely to progress onto arthrosis. In the realm of foot surgery, there is a concept that primary fusion be considered with significant comminution of certain joints, such as with severely comminuted calcaneal fractures.[51,52] Primary fusion of Lisfranc's ligamentous dislocations have also been treated with primary fusion, with results similar to that of those that undergo internal fixation, in a single

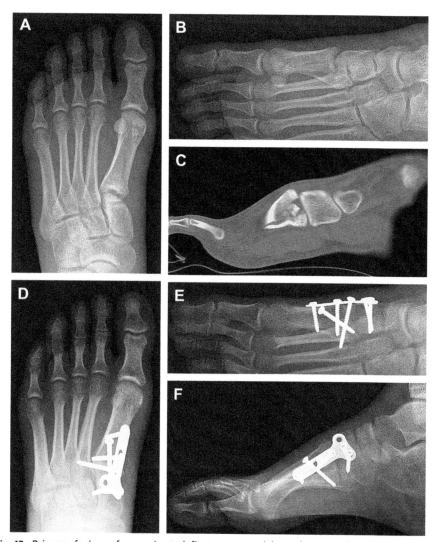

Fig. 12. Primary fusion of comminuted first metatarsal base fracture. (*A, B*) Preoperative injury radiographs demonstrating intra-articular fracture of first metatarsal base. (*C*). Computed tomography identifying comminuted intra-articular fracture. (*D–F*) Postoperative healed radiographs of primary fusion of first TMT joint (lapidus) with a dorsomedial plate. In this clinical situation, Lisfranc's ligament is secondarily stabilized with a temporary screw through the plate extending to the second metatarsal base.

prospective, randomized, controlled study.[53–55] Comminuted intra-articular fractures of the first metatarsal base may be treated with a primary fusion to avoid "inevitable" arthrosis, although specific guidelines do not dictate what degree of comminution should warrant primary fusion. Clearly, this is an area of future investigation. It should be recognized that the fixation needs of a fusion in the setting of comminution further support plate fixation (**Fig. 12**). Additionally, One should consider the stability of the Lisfranc's ligament in the context of a Lisfranc's fracture and address any instability that may concomitantly exist.

LAPIDUS WITH EARLY WEIGHTBEARING PROGRAM

The Lapidus Bunionectomy may be used in conjunction with an early postoperative weightbearing program.[7,13–15] Most retrospective studies involving the Lapidus have used a nonweightbearing postoperative protocol, and this is likely because of the early inexperience with the procedure resulting in fixation failure and subsequent nonunion. In more recent years, the overall rate of nonunion has been considered to be <10%, with a recent study showing a 5.3% nonunion rate in 227 feet.[56] Although early weightbearing is not an entirely new concept, and four published studies (level IV) show that fusion rates from 89% to 100% may be achieved with early weightbearing protocols, similar rates are reported in the literature with nonweightbearing protocols.[7,13–15] The studies using an early weightbearing protocol typically used screw fixation and an initial period of nonweightbearing followed by a progressive protected weightbearing. As part of a multicenter retrospective review study, the author reviewed his isolated Lapidus procedures that underwent an early weightbearing program (20 feet) (Blitz N, unpublished data, 2009). Crossed screw fixation with two or three solid-bore screws were used (as described earlier in this issue) and a 100% union rate was identified. In this initial investigation with the protocol, an early weightbearing program was not instituted in smokers, "elderly" with osteoporotic bone, neuropathic patients, or obese patients. The author is not advocating widespread use of the protocol, and clearly experience with Lapidus and its complications are critical to success. Nonetheless, it is clear that further studies comparing nonweightbearing protocols with early weightbearing protocols in a prospective, randomized, controlled study are the next logical steps.

SUMMARY

Although the use of the Lapidus in bunion surgery is well supported in the literature, surgeons have been expanding its indications to manage a variety of disorders affecting the foot. As more surgeons continue to gain experience with the procedure, additional studies will emerge, further supporting its versatility in the realm of foot surgery.

REFERENCES

1. Albrecht GH. The pathology and treatment of hallux valgus. Russk Vrach 1911;10: 14–9.
2. Kleinberg S. Operative cure of Hallux valgus and bunions. Am J Surg 1932;15: 98–108.
3. Truslow W. Metatarsus primus varus or hallux valgus? J Bone Joint Surg 1925;7: 75–81.
4. Lapidus PW. Operative correction of the metatarsus varus primus in hallux valgus. Surg Gynecol Obstet 1934;58:183–91.

5. Lapidus PW. A quarter century of experience with the operative correction of the metatarsus varus in hallux valgus. Bull Hosp Joint Dis 1956;17:404–21.
6. Lapidus PW. The author's bunion operation from 1931 to 1959. Clin Orthop 1960; 16:119–35.
7. Sangeorzan B, Hansen S. Modified Lapidus procedure for hallux valgus. Foot Ankle 1989;9(6):262–6.
8. Bierman RA, Christensen JC, Johnson CH. Biomechanics of the first ray. Part III. Consequences of Lapidus arthrodesis on peroneus longus function: a three-dimensional kinematic analysis in a cadaver model. J Foot Ankle Surg 2001; 40(3):125–31.
9. Avino A, Patel S, Hamilton GA, et al. The effect of the Lapidus arthrodesis on the medial longitudinal arch: a radiographic review. J Foot Ankle Surg 2008;47(6):510–4.
10. Ray RG, Ching RP, Christensen JC, et al. Biomechanical analysis of the first metatarsocuneiform arthrodesis. J Foot Ankle Surg 1998;37(5):376–85.
11. McInnes B, Bouche R. Critical evaluation of the modified Lapidus procedure. J Foot Ankle Surg 2001;40(2):71–90.
12. Catanzariti AR, Mendicino RW, Lee MS, et al. The modified Lapidus arthrodesis: a retrospective analysis. J Foot Ankle Surg 1999;38(5):322–32.
13. Bednarz PA, Manoli A 2nd. Modified Lapidus procedure for the treatment of hypermobile hallux valgus. Foot Ankle Int 2000;21(10):816–21.
14. Clark HR, Veith RG, Hansen ST Jr. Adolescent bunions treated by the modified Lapidus procedure. Bull Hosp Jt Dis Orthop Inst 1987;47(2):109–22.
15. Myerson M, Allon S, McGarvey W. Metatarsocuneiform arthrodesis for management of hallux valgus and metatarsus primus varus. Foot Ankle 1992;13(3):107–15.
16. Kopp FJ, Patel MM, Levine DS, et al. The modified Lapidus procedure for hallux valgus: a clinical and radiographic analysis. Foot Ankle Int 2005;26(11):913–7.
17. Rink-Brüne O. Lapidus arthrodesis for management of hallux valgus–a retrospective review of 106 cases. J Foot Ankle Surg 2004;43(5):290–5.
18. Coetzee JC, Wickum D. The Lapidus procedure: a prospective cohort outcome study. Foot Ankle Int 2004;25(8):526–31.
19. Popelka S, Vavrík P, Hromádka R, et al. [Our results of the Lapidus procedure in patients with hallux valgus deformity]. Acta Chir Orthop Traumatol Cech 2008; 75(4):271–6 [in Czech].
20. Popelka S, Vavrík P, Hromádka R, et al. [Lapidus procedure in patients with rheumatoid arthritis–short-term results]. Z Orthop Unfall 2008;146(1):80–5 [in German].
21. Baravarian B, Briskin GB, Burns P. Lapidus bunionectomy: arthrodesis of the first metatarsocuneiform joint. Clin Podiatr Med Surg 2004;21(1):97–111.
22. Neylon TA, Johnson BA, Laroche RA. Use of the lapidus bunionectomy in first ray insufficiency. Clin Podiatr Med Surg 2001;18(2):365–75.
23. Hansen ST Jr. Hallux valgus surgery. Morton and Lapidus were right! Clin Podiatr Med Surg 1996;13(3):347–54.
24. Kim JY, Park JS, Hwang SK, et al. Mobility changes of the first ray after hallux valgus surgery: clinical results after proximal metatarsal chevron osteotomy and distal soft tissue procedure. Foot Ankle Int 2008;29(5):468–72.
25. Myerson MS, Badekas A. Hypermobility of the first ray. Foot Ankle Clin 2000;5(3): 469–84.
26. Myerson M. Metatarsocuneiform arthrodesis for treatment of hallux valgus and metatarsus primus varus. Orthopedics 1990;13(9):1025–31.
27. Johnson KA, Kile TA. Hallux valgus due to cuneiform-metatarsal instability. J South Orthop Assoc 1994;3(4):273–82.

28. Hansen ST. Functional reconstruction of the foot and ankle. Philadelphia: Lippincott Williams & Wilkins; 2000.

29. Roling BA, Christensen JC, Johnson CH. Biomechanics of the first ray. Part IV: the effect of selected medial column arthrodeses. A three-dimensional kinematic analysis in a cadaver model. J Foot Ankle Surg 2002;41(5):278–85.

30. Faber FW, Kleinrensink GJ, Verhoog MW, et al. Mobility of the first tarsometatarsal joint in relation to hallux valgus deformity: anatomical and biomechanical aspects. Foot Ankle Int 1999;20(10):651–6.

31. Faber FW, Mulder PG, Verhaar JA. Role of first ray hypermobility in the outcome of the Hohmann and the Lapidus procedure. A prospective, randomized trial involving one hundred and one feet. J Bone Joint Surg Am 2004;86-A(3):486–95.

32. Coughlin MJ, Jones CP. Hallux valgus and first ray mobility. A prospective study. J Bone Joint Surg Am 2007;89(9):1887–98.

33. Coughlin MJ, Jones CP, Viladot R, et al. Hallux valgus and first ray mobility: a cadaveric study. Foot Ankle Int 2004;25(8):537–44.

34. Rush SM, Christensen JC, Johnson CH. Biomechanics of the first ray. Part II: Metatarsus primus varus as a cause of hypermobility. A three-dimensional kinematic analysis in a cadaver model. J Foot Ankle Surg 2000;39(2):68–77.

35. Blitz NM. Current concepts in medial column hypermobility. Podiatry Today 2005; 18:68–79.

36. Blitz NM. Use of the first ray splay test to assess transverse plane instability before first metatarsocuneiform fusion. J Foot Ankle Surg 2006;45(6):441–3.

37. Perez HR, Reber LK, Christensen JC. The effect of frontal plane position on first ray motion: forefoot locking mechanism. Foot Ankle Int 2008;29(1):72–6.

38. Grebing BR, Coughlin MJ. Evaluation of Morton's theory of second metatarsal hypertrophy. J Bone Joint Surg Am 2004;86-A(7):1375–86.

39. Morton DJ. Hypermobility of the first metatarsal bone; the interlinking factor between metatarsalgia and longitudinal arch strains. J Bone Joint Surg 1928; 10:187–96.

40. Morton DJ. The human foot: its evolution, physiology and functional disorders. Morningside Heights (NY): Columbia University Press; 1935.

41. Cohen BE, Ogden F. Medial column procedures in the acquired flatfoot deformity. Foot Ankle Clin 2007;12(2):287–99.

42. Sizensky JA, Marks RM. Medial-sided bony procedures: why, what, and how? Foot Ankle Clin 2003;8(3):539–62.

43. Hiller L, Pinney SJ. Surgical treatment of acquired flatfoot deformity: what is the state of practice among academic foot and ankle surgeons in 2002? Foot Ankle Int 2003;24(9):701–5.

44. Thompson IM, Bohay DR, Anderson JG. Fusion rate of first tarsometatarsal arthrodesis in the modified Lapidus procedure and flatfoot reconstruction. Foot Ankle Int 2005;26(9):698–703.

45. Fuhrmann RA. Arthrodesis of the first tarsometatarsal joint for correction of the advanced splayfoot accompanied by a hallux valgus. Oper Orthop Traumatol 2005;17(2):195–210.

46. Bevilacqua NJ, Rogers LC, Wrobel JS, et al. Restoration and preservation of first metatarsal length using the distraction scarf osteotomy. J Foot Ankle Surg 2008; 47(2):96–102.

47. Oznur A, Alpaslan AM. Lengthening of short great toe and correction of all lesser toe deformities by distraction-lengthening. Foot Ankle Int 2003;24(4):345–8.

48. Takakura Y, Tanaka Y, Fujii T, et al. Lengthening of short great toes by callus distraction. J Bone Joint Surg Br 1997;79(6):955–8.

49. Hamilton GA, Mullins S, Schuberth JM, et al. Revision lapidus arthrodesis: rate of union in 17 cases. J Foot Ankle Surg 2007;46(6):447–50.
50. Coetzee JC, Resig SG, Kuskowski M, et al. The Lapidus procedure as salvage after failed surgical treatment of hallux valgus: a prospective cohort study. J Bone Joint Surg Am 2003;85-A(1):60–5.
51. Huefner T, Thermann H, Geerling J, et al. Primary subtalar arthrodesis of calcaneal fractures. Foot Ankle Int 2001;22(1):9–14.
52. Huang PJ, Huang HT, Chen TB, et al. Open reduction and internal fixation of displaced intra-articular fractures of the calcaneus. J Trauma 2002;52(5):946–50.
53. Coetzee JC, Ly TV. Treatment of primarily ligamentous Lisfranc joint injuries: primary arthrodesis compared with open reduction and internal fixation. Surgical technique. J Bone Joint Surg Am 2007;89:122–7.
54. Ly TV, Coetzee JC. Treatment of primarily ligamentous Lisfranc joint injuries: primary arthrodesis compared with open reduction and internal fixation. A prospective, randomized study. J Bone Joint Surg Am 2006;88(3):514–20.
55. Mulier T, Reynders P, Dereymaeker G, et al. Severe Lisfrancs injuries: primary arthrodesis or ORIF? Foot Ankle Int 2002;23(10):902–5.
56. Patel S, Ford LA, Etcheverry J, et al. Modified lapidus arthrodesis: rate of nonunion in 227 cases. J Foot Ankle Surg 2004;43(1):37–42.

Optimizing Outcomes in Bunion Surgery

Zachary M. Haas, DPM

KEYWORDS

- Bunion • Hallux valgus • Surgery • Stability • Alignment
- Correction

A plethora of surgical approaches and procedures for deformities of the first ray have been described over the past 100 years. Although these techniques vary, they are based on the principle of anatomic restoration. Understanding the anatomy of the first ray and its biomechanical relationship to the foot and ankle are paramount in the evaluation and treatment of hallux valgus. The underlying goal of treatment not only is directed toward anatomic correction but also toward treatment based on an understanding of the cause and maintaining long-term correction.

With more than a 100 different surgical procedures described for the correction of hallux valgus, it seems difficult to determine which technique to use for any given patient. Many factors must be considered in selecting the appropriate procedure to achieve excellent long-term results. Despite various soft tissue and osseous surgical procedures and anatomic variations of each patient, the principles of anatomic restoration and stability remain consistent. These principles are eminent in achieving successful surgical outcomes.

Rush and colleagues[1] demonstrated normalization of the first ray mobility by restoring the anatomy of the first metatarsal, which in essence improves the efficiency of the plantar aponeurosis. Coughlin and Smith[2] demonstrated that surgical correction of the hallux valgus angle and the first-second intermetatarsal angle (IMA), even without a first tarsometatarsal joint arthrodesis, decreases mobility of the first ray. Maintenance of correction seems to reflect the stability of the first ray, and Coughlin and colleagues[3] believe this "stability may be a function of first ray alignment and the plantar aponeurosis." This article focuses on using various techniques and surgical adjuncts to optimize not only immediate postoperative results but also long-term maintenance of correction. This is accomplished through restoring anatomic alignment, imparting first ray stability, meticulous surgical technique, and accounting for other causes that may contribute to first ray instability.

FIRST METATARSOPHALANGEAL JOINT SOFT TISSUE ADJUNCTS

Various contractures and laxities of ligaments and tendons may be the initiating cause or the result of foot and ankle deformities. Nonetheless, particular attention must be

Albuquerque Associated Podiatrists, 121 Sycamore Street NE, Albuquerque, NM 87106, USA
E-mail address: drzhaas@gmail.com

Clin Podiatr Med Surg 26 (2009) 443–457
doi:10.1016/j.cpm.2009.03.006
0891-8422/09/$ – see front matter © 2009 Elsevier Inc. All rights reserved.

podiatric.theclinics.com

directed to restore appropriate soft tissue balance to achieve desirable results. The main soft tissue constraints in achieving anatomic correction of hallux valgus deformities at the level of the first metatarsophalangeal joint are attenuation of the medial structures and contracture of the lateral anatomy.

Once the skin incision and initial soft tissue dissection are accomplished, visualization is achieved of the first metatarsophalangeal joint capsule. Various capsulotomies have been described, including a dorsal longitudinal capsulotomy, a medial longitudinal capsulotomy, a vertical capsulotomy, and an inverted L-shaped capsulotomy with a proximal and dorsal apex or a distal and dorsal apex. A capsulorrhaphy with a longitudinal capsulotomy allows surgeons to impart a supination and varus correction of the hallux. A capsulorrhaphy with a vertical medial capsulotomy allows surgeons to medialize the hallux in the transverse plane. An inverted L-shaped capsulotomy allows surgeons versatility in terms of soft tissue correction in the frontal and transverse planes.

When performing a capsulotomy along with dissection for the planned osteotomy or arthrodesis, many investigators state the importance of soft tissue preservation in maintaining the periosteum at the neck of the first metatarsal head.[4–7] This meticulous dissection aids in preventing the incidence of avascular necrosis, as the blood supply enters at this level.[7] Malal and colleagues[8] evaluated the vascular supply of the first metatarsal head that is supplied by branches of the first dorsal metatarsal, first plantar metatarsal, and medial plantar arteries. They showed that although the first dorsal metatarsal artery is the prominent artery, all three arteries form a plexus and enter at the plantar lateral aspect of the metatarsal neck. This suggests that medial and dorsal capsulotomies are safe with regard to the main vascular supply of the first metatarsal head, but careful attention must be directed if creating a distal first metatarsal osteotomy or a lateral first metatarsophalangeal joint soft tissue release that is in close approximation to the metatarsal neck.

In pathologic hallux valgus, the sesamoids are deviated laterally, leading to a mechanical advantage of the lateral joint structures, which subsequently become a primary deforming force potentiating the abducted position of the hallux.[9] Releasing the lateral soft tissue contractures removes this underlying deforming force and allows for mobilization of the first ray with respect to the sesamoid apparatus. This mobilization is important in restoring proper positioning of the sesamoids along with the plantar aponeurosis. Sarrafian[10] stated the importance of the plantar aponeurosis alignment in providing stability to the first ray. Oda[11] used tibial sesamoid position (TSP) to analyze outcomes of a modified Lapidus arthrodesis. The TSP was assessed relative to the first metatarsal head on a scale of 1 to 7, with a position of 4 representing the tibial sesamoid being a midline alignment. The study demonstrated that TSP correlated with the amount of correction, as satisfactory cases corrected a mean of 5.5 positions and undercorrected cases corrected a mean of 2.5 positions.

First interspace dissection along with releasing the plantar lateral soft tissue contractures have been described by various approaches.[4–7] Coughlin and Mann[4] described a specific sequence of release: fibular sesamoidal ligament transection, adductor hallucis tendon transection or transfer, transverse metatarsal ligament transection, and lateral capsule perforation. Releasing those structures aides in mobilizing the hallux and the sesamoid apparatus to achieve a reducible hallux and relocate the first metatarsal over the sesamoid complex. This relocation is essential to decreasing the potential of a recurrent hallux valgus.[4] After releasing the fibular sesamoidal ligament, inspection should be performed of the fibular sesamoid to assess degenerative changes. The fibular sesamoid should be preserved, except in cases of significant degenerative changes, to reduce the incidence of hallux varus and tibial sesamoid overload. The adductor hallucis tendon may be mobilized and transected, removed to prevent possible reattachment and recurrence,[7] or transferred to the first metatarsal head.[12] Martinez-Nova and colleagues[12] showed there was no statistical significance when comparing an adductor hallucis tendon transfer versus a transection with regards to the first-second IMA, hallux abductus angle, or tibial sesamoid position. Coughlin and Mann[4] describe a perforation technique with subsequent tearing of the lateral capsule by manual manipulation of the hallux. They state the importance in providing a lateral stabilizing force at the first metatarsophalangeal joint and reducing the risk for postoperative hallux varus.

After performing a medial capsulotomy and a lateral soft tissue release, along with an osseous procedure to realign the first ray, the final step in balancing the soft tissues at the level of the first metatarsophalangeal joint is repair of the medial capsule. After osseous realignment of the first metatarsal and anatomic restoration of the hallux, parallel to the lesser digits in the transverse plane and with the nail parallel to the weight-bearing surface in the frontal plane, redundant medial or dorsal capsule is removed to allow for adequate tension and apposition. An inverted L-shaped capsulotomy, with the dorsal limb parallel to the extensor hallucis longus at the level of the first metatarsal head and the vertical limb perpendicular to the weight-bearing surface at the level of the metatarsal head, allows surgeons to remove redundancy medially to correct for transverse plane laxity and dorsally to correct for frontal plane laxity. As an adjunct to ensure proper positioning of the sesamoid apparatus with the use of soft tissue rebalancing, surgeons may use a hemostat placed at the apex of the inverted L-shaped capsulotomy (**Fig. 1**) and tension the capsule under fluoroscopic guidance (**Fig. 2**). This allows direct visualization of the sesamoid position to potentially avoid overtightening the medial structures and prevent a peaking tibial sesamoid and the possibility of hallux varus. This also allows surgeons to assess for undercorrection to avoid a recurrent hallux valgus deformity. Once the sesamoids are in the desired position, the redundant medial or dorsal capsule is excised and the remaining capsule

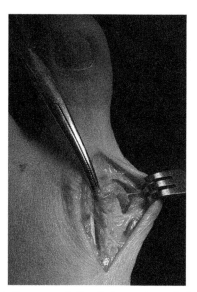

Fig. 1. Using a hemostat at the apex of the first metatarsophalangeal joint, capsulotomy allows surgeons to adequately tension and align the sesamoid complex and capsule.

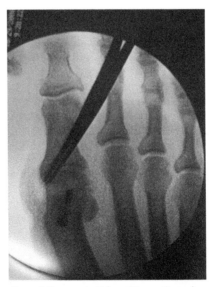

Fig. 2. Flouroscopic evaluation of the sesamoid position using a hemostat to apply tension at the apex of the first metatarsophalangeal joint capsulotomy.

subsequently repaired with absorbable suture in the corrected position. An isolated longitudinal medial capsulorrhaphy and a vertical capsulorrhaphy also have been described as an adjunct to osseous correction.[4–7,13] When using a longitudinal capsulorrhaphy a Kocher clamp can be used to grasp the plantar aspect of the capsulotomy and apply dorsal tension to facilitate realignment of the sesamoid complex in the frontal plane. When performing a vertical capsulorrhaphy, a clamp again may be used to grasp the distal aspect of the capsulotomy and apply proximal tension to appropriately align the hallux in the transverse plane. The subsequent redundant tissue is again excised and the capsule is reapproximated with absorbable suture material.

An equinus deformity at the level of the ankle joint should be assessed and addressed in conjunction with a hallux valgus deformity. Coughlin and Mann[4] state the importance of correcting the foot to a plantigrade position before repairing a hallux valgus deformity to prevent an unsatisfactory postoperative outcome. Hanson[14] describes a pathologic planovalgus deformity secondary to a disruption of the normal biomechanics caused by a gastrocnemius contracture or equinus deformity. This may lead to supination or elevation of the first metatarsal with a resultant hallux valgus deformity. Silfverskiold[15] described a method to evaluate and differentiate gastrocnemius equinus from gastrocsoleal equinus. With patients seated and an examiner positioning the hindfoot, midfoot, and forefoot in neutral position, the amount of dorsiflexion at the level of the ankle joint is assessed with the knee extended and the knee bent. Hansen[14] describes this technique as mimicking the locked position of a normal foot during late stance. In the presence of gastrocnemius equinus, the ankle cannot dorsiflex to a neutral position with the knee straight but can dorsiflex between 5° and 35° with the knee extended.[14] If ankle dorsiflexion is limited with the knee extended and the knee flexed, the diagnosis is a gastrocsoleal equinus or an osseous ankle equinus. Lateral weight-bearing radiographs of the foot and ankle with the knee straight are useful in evaluating osseous ankle equinus along with detecting an incongruity in the talar-first metatarsal line associated with a gastrocne-mius equinus.[14]

Treatment for an equinus deformity is directed toward lengthening the contracted muscle tendon unit. Nonoperative modalities consist of stretching, physical therapy, casting, and night splints. Ballistic and static stretching exercises have shown to significantly improve ankle dorsiflexion range of motion.[16] When nonoperative treat-ment fails, surgical lengthening is performed. Various techniques have been reported in the literature for a gastrocnemius recession. Blitz and Rush[17] describe a technique called a gastrocnemius intramuscular aponeurotic recession that allows for isolated lengthening of the gastrocnemius, avoidance of the sural nerve, and avoidance of weakening the gastrocnemius complex by preserving the gastrocnemius insertion. This procedure is performed with patients supine and leg elevated. A medial longitu-dinal incision is made at the midsubstance of the gastrocnemius muscle belly with close attention directed toward avoiding the saphenous nerve and vein during soft tissue dissection. After soft tissue dissection, the crural fascia is identified and incised in line with the skin incision. The gastrocsoleal interval is identified and the gastrocne-mius aponeurosis is isolated and transected in a transverse manner with tension applied through extension at the knee joint and dorsiflexion at the ankle joint. The underlying muscle belly is appreciated and a gap in the aponeurosis of 1 to 3 cm should be expected. Closure subsequently is performed in layers to include the crural fascia and the skin. Rush and colleagues[18] describe performing a high gastrocnemius recession with low associated morbidity. They evaluated 126 patients who had no residual decrease in muscle strength, gait disturbance, or overcorrection.

OSSEOUS ADJUNCTS

Proper first ray osseous alignment and stability lead to maintenance of correction and excellent subjective and objective results.[2,19,20] These principles are accomplished with selecting the appropriate procedure for a given patient along with the proper execution of that procedure. Patient demographics and convalescence along with subjective, objective, and radiographic parameters must be weighed equally. Histor-ically, the treatment of mild to moderate hallux valgus deformity entails several distal first metatarsal osteotomies and moderate to severe deformities are treated with prox-imal first metatarsal osteotomies or a first tarsometatarsal joint arthrodesis. Based on procedure selection, the osteotomy or arthrodesis may allow correction of deformity in the transverse, sagittal, or frontal planes.

After a proper release of the soft tissue constraints at the level of the first metatar-sophalangeal joint, attention is directed to the medial eminence of the first metatarsal head. When performing a distal first metatarsal osteotomy, resection of the medial eminence allows a flat surface for the planned osteotomy. The resection can be per-formed with a chisel, an osteotome, or a saw. The medial eminence may be cut from distal to proximal or dorsal to plantar to ensure a smooth transition with the first meta-tarsal metaphysis. Careful attention must be directed to avoid the sesamoid articula-tion, with the exostectomy performed in the direction of dorsal medial to plantar lateral. An aggressive resection of the medial eminence may result in medial sublux-ation of the tibial sesamoid that may lead to hallux varus or sesamoid pathology. When performing a proximal first metatarsal osteotomy or first tarsometatarsal joint arthrodesis, surgeons should resect the medial eminence after correction of the defor-mity is achieved. With correction of the first-second IMA through a proximal first ray procedure, the sesamoid complex realigns, potentially altering the amount of neces-sary resection of the medial eminence. A subtle rotation of the first metatarsal head may occur after correction of first ray deformity, leading to malrotation if the exostectomy initially is performed.[7]

Although the literature describes many distal metatarsal osteotomy techniques, the most common is the Austin or chevron bunionectomy. This bunionectomy uses a V-shaped osteotomy orientated from medial to lateral with a distally based apex centered in the first metatarsal head and approximately 8 mm proximal to the articular surface.[6] The plantar arm of the osteotomy should not be angled vertical as this could lead to dorsal instability followed by malunion.[6] To decrease the incidence of avascular necrosis at the first metatarsal head, the plantar arm should exit proximal to the plantar lateral first metatarsophalangeal joint capsular attachment to avoid disruption of the major site of first metatarsal head vascular inflow.[8] The angulation of the osteotomy may be modified to accommodate deformity in the sagittal plane and with regard to the metatarsal length. An apical axis guide uses a Kirschner wire to assist surgeons in performing an osteotomy in the desired angle and plane.[21] When performing the osteotomy, the sagittal or oscillating saw should remain in the same plane created by the Kirschner wire to prevent malrotation. When using the apical axis guide for correction, it is useful to use the second metatarsal as a reference.

In correcting a stable elevatus first ray deformity or a second metatarsal overload, the apical axis guide may be directed from dorsal medial to plantar lateral.[21] Once the osteotomy is complete, this angulation allows the capital fragment to achieve a plantarflexed position when transposed laterally. In correcting a short first metatarsal or a second metatarsal overload, the apical axis guide may be directed from proximal medial to distal lateral. Once the osteotomy is complete, the capital fragment is transposed distal and lateral. If shortening the first ray is desired, the axis guide may be directed from distal medial to proximal lateral in the first metatarsal head.

Once a distal first metatarsal osteotomy is completed, the capital fragment is transposed laterally to reduce the relative first-second IMA along with accommodating for possible elevatus of the first ray, shortening of the first ray, or second metatarsal overload. When attempting to lengthen the first ray (with the osteotomy angulated from proximal medial to distal lateral), the capital fragment may be constrained by the lateral capsule of the first metatarsophalangeal joint. When encountering this constraint, surgeons may use a Freer elevator or an osteotome within the osteotomy and provide a medial distracting force to mobilize the capital fragment further. The amount of transposition is determined in many ways by various investigators. Badwey and colleagues[22] concluded that the capital fragment could be transposed 6 mm in men and 5 mm in women. Myerson[6] describes limiting the transposition to less than one third of the first metatarsal width at the level of the metatarsal neck. This limit helps to avoid the possibilities of avascular necrosis and instability. Cooke (Robert Cooke, DPM, personal communication, November 2005) uses a radiographic technique to ensure proper alignment of the first metatarsal head with respect to the sesamoid apparatus. On weight-bearing anterior-posterior foot preoperative radiographs, the distance in millimeters is measured from the lateral aspect of the first metatarsal head to the lateral aspect of the fibular sesamoid (**Fig. 3**). A proper release of the soft tissue constraints on the first metatarsal head and a first metatarsal distal osteotomy allows a reference to laterally transpose the first metatarsal head. Intraoperatively, surgeons may directly measure the amount of capital fragment lateral translation with a ruler. The ruler measures the distance from the medial aspect of the transposed capital fragment to the medial aspect of the remaining overhanging edge of the proximal fragment (**Fig. 4**). This technique allows surgeons to achieve proper positioning of the capital fragment relative to the sesamoid complex, which contributes to the overall stability and maintenance of correction of the first

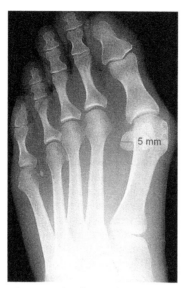

Fig. 3. A weight-bearing anterior-posterior foot radiograph is used to measure the preoperative distance in millimeters from the lateral aspect of the first metatarsal head to the lateral aspect of the fibular sesamoid.

ray.[11,19,20] Another technique uses the preoperative first-second IMA to determine the amount of lateral translation. Jahss and colleagues[23] and Sarrafian and colleagues[24] showed a 1° first-second IMA correction with each 1 mm of lateral translation of the capital fragment. After a surgeon performs a distal first metatarsal bunionectomy and an initially unrecognized instability of the first ray exists after fixation, a distal suture or a lag screw between the first and second metatarsals can be used, a technique described by Myerson.[7]

For the treatment of moderate to severe hallux valgus deformity, several proximal bunionectomies have been proposed with accompanying debate regarding optimal necessity and efficacy.[25] One of these procedures is the modified Lapidus arthrodesis, initially described by Albrecht in 1911[26] and later popularized by Lapidus in

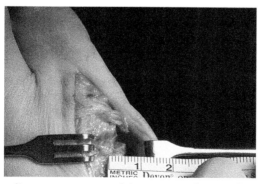

Fig. 4. Intraoperative direct measurement of the amount of capital fragment translation by measuring the distance from the medial aspect of the transposed capital fragment to the medial aspect of the remaining overhanging edge of the proximal fragment.

1934.[27] There have been several advocates for performing a modified Lapidus arthrodesis for the correction of hallux valgus. Several indications have been described, including transverse or sagittal plane instability, a medially orientated first tarsometatarsal joint, and a moderate to severe first-second IMA.[4,6,7,19] Instability of the first ray may be demonstrated on clinical or radiographic examination. Clinical examination includes stabilizing the lesser metatarsals in maximum dorsiflexion and manipulating the first metatarsal head into maximum dorsiflexion with the forefoot relaxed.[14] Hansen[14] defines hypermobility as first ray elevation greater than 5 to 8 mm with this technique. Other correlating findings are keratosis formation under the lesser metatarsal heads and the plantar medial aspect of the hallux interphalangeal joint, a dorsal first tarsometatarsal joint exostosis, limited first metatarsophalangeal joint motion, synovitis of the second metatarsophalangeal joint or the second tarso-metatarsal joint, tenderness of the subsecond metatarsal head, instability or subluxa-tion at the second metatarsophalangeal joint, medial arch pain, and shoe wear difficulties.[14] Radiographic criteria include plantar gaping at the first tarsometatarsal joint, hypertrophy of the second metatarsal, enlarged second metatarsal head, subluxation or dislocation at the second or third metatarsophalangeal joints, widening of the second metatarsophalangeal joint, second or third tarsometatarsal joint arthrosis, first metatarsal osteoporosis, and elevation of the first metatarsal with respect to the lesser metatarsals.[14,20,28–31] Physicians also must assess various hind-foot abnormalities, as these may be the cause or an exacerbating factor of first ray instability. Blackwood and colleagues[32] demonstrated with statistical significance that motion of the metatarsals in the sagittal plane is increased with hindfoot valgus. Increased pronation may be secondary to gastrocnemius equinus or posterior tibial tendon weakness or dysfunction.[14] These pathologies must be addressed to ensure stabilization of the first ray, thus maintaining long-term correction.

A Lapidus arthrodesis corrects for a large first-second IMA and uneven weight distribution at the level of the metatarsal heads and imparts stability to the first ray. This stability is paramount to maintaining long-term correction.[19] Stability of the first ray is imparted through adequate transverse plane position,[1,2,33] adequate frontal plane position,[34] and internal fixation of the first tarsometatarsal joint.[28] Positioning is achieved after adequate preparation of the first tarsometatarsal joint. Myerson[7] describes the key to joint débridement is restraint because minimal sub-chondral bone should be removed after complete removal of the articular carti-lage. This prevents unnecessary shortening and maintains structural support at the level of the joint interface. Perforation subsequently is performed of the sub-chondral bone using a fish scaling technique with an osteotome and a mallet or by fenestration with a drill bit or Kirschner wire. The fish scaling technique is preferred to help prevent the incidence of thermal necrosis. Correct positioning is performed in all three anatomic planes to ensure adequate angular correction and stability. The transverse plane is evaluated by reducing the first-second IMA and ensuring appropriate position of the sesamoid apparatus. The sagittal plane is assessed by ensuring the declination of the first metatarsal is congruent with the lesser metatarsals. Perez and colleagues[34] demonstrated the relevance of frontal plane position on first ray stability. They demonstrated that an everted posi-tion of the first ray resulted in maximum sagittal plane mobility. Positioning the first ray is accomplished with rotation and translation at the level of the metatarsal base. Myerson[7] described a maneuver of dorsiflexing the hallux, squeezing the first metatarsal to the second metatarsal, and impacting the first tarsometatarsal joint. This technique forces the first metatarsal into slight plantarflexion, reduces the IMA, and apposes the first tarsometatarsal joint. Once position is confirmed, internal fixation is used to maintain correction and to provide compression and strength.

Although stability of the first ray usually is accomplished with anatomic positioning and a first tarsometatarsal joint arthrodesis, there are instances when the first ray remains mobile despite this procedure. An intraoperative adjunct to evaluate any residual mobility is to access the amount of transverse and sagittal plane first ray stability after fixation of the first tarsometatarsal joint. Ford and Hamilton (Lawrence Ford, DPM, and Graham Hamilton, DPM, personal communication, July 2005) routinely stress the first ray, after adequate internal fixation of the first tarsometatarsal joint, in the transverse plane to ensure adequate stability. This technique consists of placing a finger in the first interspace and evaluating the amount of transverse plane instability between the first and second metatarsal heads. If instability is evident, surgeons must account for this issue to ensure maintenance of correction. The relationship between the first and second metatarsals and the medial and intermediate cuneiforms may explain the occasional continued instability. Various techniques have been described for addressing this instability. Hanson[35] describes a technique of inserting a screw from the base of the first metatarsal to the base of the second metatarsal to correct for a varus deformity or to provide further correction of the first-second IMA. Other techniques include an additional screw from the first metatarsal base to the intermediate cuneiform (**Fig. 5**) or from the medial cuneiform to the intermediate cuneiform (**Fig. 6**). Using the intermediate cuneiform or the second ray as an adjunct to a first tarsometatarsal joint arthrodesis may impart further stability to the first ray.

When first ray stability is present preoperatively in the setting of a moderate to severe first-second IMA, surgical correction may be performed distal to the first tarsometatarsal joint. Many first metatarsal proximal osteotomies have been described for a moderate to severe hallux valgus deformity. These include a proximal crescentic

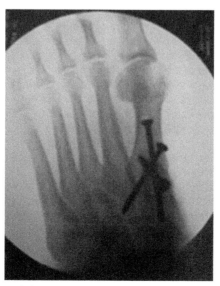

Fig. 5. When first ray instability continues to persist despite a first tarsometatarsal joint arthrodesis, a third screw may be used to stabilize the first ray from the first metatarsal base to the intermediate cuneiform.

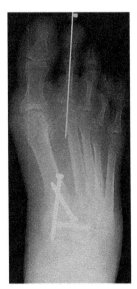

Fig. 6. When first ray instability continues to persist despite a first tarsometatarsal joint arthrodesis, a third screw may be used to stabilize the first ray from the medial cuneiform to the intermediate cuneiform.

osteotomy, a closing base wedge osteotomy, an opening base wedge osteotomy, an oblique osteotomy, and a proximal chevron osteotomy. Coughlin and Smith[2] reported on a 27-month mean follow-up for 103 proximal crescentic osteotomies with a distal first metatarsophalangeal joint rebalancing. They reported 93% good to excellent results with mean American Orthopaedic Foot and Ankle Society (AOFAS) scores improving from 57 points preoperatively to 91 points postoperatively. They also associated a decrease in first ray hypermobility with surgical correction. Although a proximal crescentic osteotomy has been demonstrated to maintain the length of the first ray and impart stability,[4] others have shown an association with a dorsal malunion with subsequent limitation of the first metatarsophalangeal joint and transfer metatarsalgia.[6,36,37] A closing base wedge osteotomy has a predictable healing pattern but may lead to shortening and possibly elevation of the first ray. An opening base wedge osteotomy has been advocated to elongate the first ray, although with the risk for nonunion this procedure rarely is indicated.[6] Myerson favors a 30°oblique first metatarsal base osteotomy, as this allows early weight bearing and the ability to correct for first metatarsal shortening through the use of changing the plane of the osteotomy. His research also supports more stability to metatarsal stress loading with an oblique osteotomy than with a proximal chevron osteotomy or a crescentic osteotomy.[6] Trnka and colleagues[38] reported on the largest cohort of patients undergoing an oblique osteotomy for the correction of hallux valgus. Their study included 111 feet with significant improvements to the AOFAS scores along with correction of the hallux abductus angle and the first-second IMA. All osteotomy sites healed without a dorsal malunion but averaged 2.2 mm of first metatarsal shortening. When compared with a crescentic osteotomy, research demonstrates that a proximal chevron osteotomy has greater strength and stability and less of an incidence of associated transfer lesions.[39,40] Kim and colleagues[33] showed a statistically significant reduction in first ray dorsiflexion mobility 1 year after a proximal metatarsal chevron osteotomy and distal metatarsophalangeal joint rebalancing. They used a modified Klaue device on 82 patients who had a mean dorsiflexion mobility of the first ray decreasing from 6.8 mm to 3.2 mm.

Assessing the relative length of the first ray also is paramount in determining the optimal surgical procedure. A short first ray may be associated with lesser metatarsalgia, keratosis under the second metatarsal head, and cortical thickening of the second metatarsal with or without lesser digit deformities. The first metatarsal head and associated sesamoids should carry one third of the body weight, with the lesser metatarsal heads distributing the remainder of the weight equally.[13] This weight distribution is essential for normal gait mechanics and must be restored in patients undergoing surgical repair for a pathologic first ray deformity. If the first metatarsal declination angle is 25°, Jahss and colleagues[23] demonstrated for each 1 mm of metatarsal shortening a corresponding 0.42-mm elevation of the metatarsal exists. Thus, for each metatarsal osteotomy surgeons must compensate for this potential uneven weight distribution with techniques related to translation, lengthening, and angulation. The thickness of the saw blade accounts for 1 to 2 mm of shortening and an additional 1 mm may occur from heat necrosis and bony resorption.[6] As discussed previously, when performing a distal metatarsal osteotomy, surgeons may direct the osteotomy from proximal medial to distal lateral to lengthen a short first metatarsal or accommodate for the bone loss associated with using a saw blade. Lengthening also may be accomplished with a proximal bunionectomy. Hansen[13] describes a first tarsometatarsal joint arthrodesis with the use of a lamina spreader after preparation for fusion. The joint is distracted until normal length is achieved, this distance is measured, and a tricortical iliac crest bone graft is used and modeled to fit the gap. Lengthening the first ray may be limited by the restriction of motion at the first metatarsophalangeal joint. In these instances, along with significantly elongated lesser metatarsals, an adjunct may include shortening osteotomies of the lesser metatarsals to restore an anatomic metatarsal parabola.

The role of the proximal articular set angle, or distal metatarsal articular angle (DMAA), in hallux valgus pathology is controversial. An increase in the DMAA has been attributed to general adaptation of the distal first metatarsal articular surface, an adaptation that may result from longstanding hallux valgus.[41] This angle has been described as the angle formed between a line perpendicular to the long axis of the first metatarsal and a line coincident with the functional articular cartilage of the first metatarsal head. The established range of normal values for this angle is from 0° to 8°, but radiographic appearance of the actual articular surface orientation may differ from its intraoperative visual appearance.[42] Some investigators believe this should be addressed with surgical realignment at the time of surgery[6] whereas others believe physiologic remodeling from adequate realignment of the first metatarsophalangeal joint is sufficient and superior.[13] Myerson[6] stressed the importance of adding a biplanar distal metatarsal osteotomy or a hallux phalangeal osteotomy to a distal metatarsal osteotomy when the first-second IMA is less than 14° and the DMAA is greater than 15°. He also describes combining a proximal metatarsal osteotomy and a distal closing wedge osteotomy for an increased first-second IMA and DMAA. Contrary to this method, Hansen[13] describes physiologic remodeling of the articular cartilage as superior to an osteotomy because of the risks for avascular necrosis along with adhesions and fibrosis in the associated joint capsule.

Articular cartilage functions primarily to support and distribute loads and to provide lubrication in diarthrodial joints.[43] Kaab and colleagues[44] showed that chondrocytes undergo major changes in shape and are sensitive to differences in the magnitude and duration of loads being applied. Mechanical load and hydrostatic pressure thus regulate the activity of chondrocytes and create the adaptation necessary to preserve their load-bearing function.[44] These properties suggest that adaptive changes in joints occur secondarily to repetitive force and that theoretically an increase in the DMAA would be secondary to a longstanding hallux valgus deformity. This also suggests that correction of the DMAA could be achieved through proper alignment of the hallux abductus angle without direct surgical correction of the dysfunctional DMAA.

A dysfunctional DMAA has been corrected by various techniques that realign the articular cartilage to provide a congruent and anatomically aligned joint or by correcting the alignment of the hallux with a phalangeal osteotomy. The earliest report of realigning the articular cartilage was published in 1881, when Reverdin[45] described a distal osteotomy of the first metatarsal with resection of the medial eminence and a medially based incomplete closing wedge osteotomy of the first metatarsal head. Removing a triangular wedge of bone achieves structural correction by aligning the joint surface perpendicular to the metatarsal shaft.[21] The original technique subsequently was modified by several investigators and now commonly is described as a distal L or Reverdin-Green-Laird procedure. This procedure enables the surgeon to correct an abnormal articular set angle along with an increased IMA. Another technique is described by Coughlin and Mann,[4] who recommend a biplanar medial closing wedge chevron osteotomy if valgus remains after transposition of the capital fragment. Rather than correcting an abnormal DMAA directly, Myerson[6] believes it is favorable to maintain the metatarsophalangeal joint shape and to correct the alignment with a phalangeal osteotomy. Although this preserves the joint, the forces across the metatarsophalangeal joint would remain abnormal and possibly increase the rate of recurrence.

A proximal phalangeal medial based wedge osteotomy, otherwise known as the Akin procedure, is an osseous adjunct commonly used in bunion surgery. The indications include a hallux valgus interphalangeus, a congruent metatarsophalangeal joint with an increased distal metatarsal articulation angle, or a residual lateral or hallux valgus deviation after completion of a first metatarsal osteotomy or a first tarsometatarsal joint arthrodesis with metatarsophalangeal joint rebalancing.[4,6] Coughlin and Mann correlate recurrent hallux valgus deformity and inadequate correction after a chevron procedure to a failure in recognizing an increased DMAA.[4] They stress measuring the preoperative angle and adding an Akin procedure or a medial closing wedge distal first metatarsal osteotomy if the angle is greater than 15°. The location of the proximal phalanx osteotomy should be performed at the site of maximum deformity. This deformity is evaluated through the use of preoperative radiographs. If the maximum deformity is at the proximal portion of the proximal phalanx, surgeons should make the proximal cut parallel to the base of the proximal phalanx to prevent penetration into the articular surface. When performing this osteotomy, surgeons must avoid penetrating the lateral phalangeal cortex to improve the stability of the osteotomy and maintain the first metatarsophalangeal joint capsule to potentially allow a medial capsulorrhaphy.[6] Myerson[7] described a technique to supinate the hallux when performing an Akin osteotomy. This technique uses one set of pilot holes on the proximal side of the osteotomy in line with the medial aspect of the phalangeal shaft and one set of pilot holes on the distal side of the osteotomy drilled more plantar (approximately 2 mm inferior to the proximal holes). Once the osteotomy is completed and closed, the hallux is supinated to align the two sets of holes. If these holes are drilled at a 45° angle to the planned osteotomy, they may be used to pass suture for fixation and closure. Recurrent deformities may arise when performing an isolated Akin procedure for subluxation at the level of the first metatarsophalangeal joint or an increased first-second IMA due to a failure in correcting the underlying biomechanical deformity and metatarsophalangeal joint imbalance.[4,7,46,47]

SUMMARY

The goal of fine-tuning bunion surgery is to optimize outcomes and prevent complications. These tasks can be accomplished with diligent preoperative examination and planning, appropriate surgical procedure and technique, and adequate postoperative care. Soft tissue rebalancing at the first metatarsophalangeal joint is important to freely mobilize the sesamoid apparatus for adequate positioning with respect to the first metatarsal head. This positioning leads to mechanical stability of the first ray by realignment of the plantar aponeurosis. Selecting the appropriate osseous procedure allows correction of the first-second IMA and confers the stability to the first ray. Postoperative stability to the first ray is provided through realignment in the frontal[34] and transverse planes[2,33] along with a first tarsometatarsal joint arthrodesis.[35] Appropriate sagittal plane positioning is paramount in ensuring equal weight distribution to the metatarsal heads for normal gait mechanics. The entire lower extremity, including the rearfoot and the superficial posterior muscle group, must be evaluated and addressed, as these factors may contribute to osseous malalignment and instability of the first ray. Maintenance of correction is predicated on the treatment of underlying pathology and the establishment of optimal stability and first ray alignment.

REFERENCES

1. Rush SM, Christensen JC, Johnson CH. Biomechanics of the first ray. part II: metatarsus primus varus as a cause of hypermobility. A three-dimensional kinematic analysis in a cadaver model. J Foot Ankle Surg 2000;39(2):68–77.
2. Coughlin MJ, Smith BW. Hallux valgus and first ray mobility. Surgical technique. J Bone Joint Surg Am 2008;2(90 Suppl 2 Pt):153–70.
3. Coughlin MJ, Jones CP, Viladot R, et al. Hallux valgus and first ray mobility: a cadaveric study. Foot Ankle Int 2004;25(8):537–44.
4. Coughlin MJ, Mann RA. Hallux valgus. In: Coughlin MJ, Mann RA, Saltzman CL, editors. Surgery of the foot and ankle. 8th edition. Philadelphia: Mosby Inc; 2007. p. 183–362.
5. Ruch JA, Peebles CF, Sun CA, et al. Anatomic dissection of the first metatarsophalangeal joint for hallux valgus surgery. In: Banks AS, Downey MS, Martin DE, et al, editors. McGlamry's comprehensive textbook of foot and ankle surgery. 3rd edition. Philadelphia: Lippincott Williams & Wilkins; 2001. p. 493–504.
6. Myerson MS. Hallux valgus. In: Myerson MS, editor. Foot and ankle disorders. Philadelphia: W.B. Saunders; 2000. p. 213–88.
7. Myerson MS. The hallux: hallux valgus. In: Reconstructive foot and ankle surgery. 1st edition. Philadelphia: Elsevier Inc; 2005. p. 1–86.
8. Malal JJ, Shaw-Dunn J, Kumar CS. Blood supply to the first metatarsal head and vessels at risk with a chevron osteotomy. J Bone Joint Surg Am 2007;89(9): 2018–22.
9. Martin DE, Pontious J, et al. Introduction and evaluation of hallux abducto valgus. In: Banks AS, Downey MS, Martin DE, et al, editors. McGlamry's comprehensive textbook of foot and ankle surgery. 3rd edition. Philadelphia: Lippincott Williams & Wilkins; 2001. p. 481–91.
10. Sarrafian SK. Functional characteristics of the foot and plantar aponeurosis under tibiotalar loading. Foot Ankle 1987;8(1):4–18.
11. Oda RB. Lapidus arthrodesis for management of hallux valgus—a retrospective review of 106 cases. J Foot Ankle Surg 2004;43(5):290–5.

12. Martinez-Nova A, Sanchez-Rodriguez R, Gomez-Martin B, et al. The effect of adductor tendon transposition in the modified mcbride procedure. Foot & Ankle Specialist 2008;1(5):275–9.

13. Hansen ST Jr. The dysfunctional forefoot. In: Functional reconstruction of the foot and ankle. Philadelphia: Lippencott Williams & Wilkins; 2000. p. 215–26.

14. Hansen ST Jr. Functional anatomy. In: Functional reconstruction of the foot and ankle. Philadelphia: Lippencott Williams & Wilkins; 2000. p. 17–32.

15. Silfverskiold N. Reduction of the uncrossed two-joints muscles of the leg to one-joint muscles in spastic conditions. Acta Chir Scand 1924;56:315.

16. Mahieu NN, McNair P, De Muynck M, et al. Effect of static and ballistic stretching on the muscle-tendon tissue properties. Med Sci Sports Exerc 2007;39(3):494–501.

17. Blitz NM, Rush SM. The gastrocnemius intramuscular aponeurotic recession: a simplified method of gastrocnemius recession. J Foot Ankle Surg 2007;46(2): 133–8.

18. Rush SM, Ford LA, Hamilton GA. Morbidity associated with high gastrocnemius recession: retrospective review of 126 cases. J Foot Ankle Surg 2006;45(3): 156–60.

19. Haas Z, Hamilton G, Sundstrom D, et al. Maintenance of correction of first metatarsal closing base wedge osteotomies versus modified Lapidus arthrodesis for moderate to severe hallux valgus deformity. J Foot Ankle Surg 2007;46(5): 358–65.

20. McInnes BD, Bouche RT. Critical evaluation of the modified Lapidus procedure. J Foot Ankle Surg 2001;40(2):71–90.

21. Chang TJ, et al. Distal metaphyseal osteotomies in hallux abducto valgus surgery. In: Banks AS, Downey MS, Martin DE, et al, editors. McGlamry's comprehensive textbook of foot and ankle surgery. 3rd edition. Philadelphia: Lippincott Williams & Wilkins; 2001. p. 505–27.

22. Badwey TM, Dutkowsky JP, Graves SC, et al. An anatomical basis for the degree of displacement of the distal chevron osteotomy in the treatment of hallux valgus. Foot Ankle Int 1997;18(4):213–5.

23. Jahss MH, Troy AI, Kummer F. Roentgenographic and mathematical analysis of first metatarsal osteotomies for metatarsus primus varus: a comparative study. Foot Ankle 1985;5(6):280–321.

24. Sarrafian SK. A method of predicting the degree of functional correction of the metatarsus primus varus with a distal lateral displacement osteotomy in hallux valgus. Foot Ankle 1985;5(6):322–6.

25. Mothershed RA, Catanzariti AR, Blitch EL, et al. Proximal procedures of the first ray. In: Banks AS, Downey MS, Martin DE, et al, editors. McGlamry's comprehensive textbook of foot and ankle surgery. 3rd edition. Philadelphia: Lippincott Williams & Wilkins; 2001. p. 529–56.

26. Albrecht GH. The pathology and treatment of hallux valgus. Russ Vrach 1911;10: 14–9.

27. Lapidus P. Operative correction of the metatarsus varus primus in hallux valgus. Surg Gynecol Obstet 1934;58:183–91.

28. Sangeorzan BJ, Hansen ST Jr. Modified Lapidus procedure for hallux valgus. Foot Ankle 1989;9(6):262–6.

29. Myerson M, Allon S, McGarvey W. Metatarsocuneiform arthrodesis for management of hallux valgus and metatarsus primus varus. Foot Ankle 1992;13(3): 107–15.

30. Myerson MS, Badekas A. Hypermobility of the first ray. Foot Ankle Clin 2000;5(3): 469–84.

31. Lapidus PW. Authors bunion operation from 1931–1959. Clin Orthop 1960;16: 119–35.
32. Blackwood CB, Yuen TJ, Sangeorzan BJ, et al. The midtarsal joint locking mechanism. Foot Ankle Int 2005;26(12):1074–80.
33. Kim JY, Park JS, Hwang SK, et al. Mobility changes of the first ray after hallux valgus surgery: clinical results after proximal metatarsal chevron osteotomy and distal soft tissue procedure. Foot Ankle Int 2008;29(5):468–72.
34. Perez HR, Reber LK, Christensen JC. The effect of frontal plane position on first ray motion: forefoot locking mechanism. Foot Ankle Int 2008;29(1):72–6.
35. Hansen ST. First tarsometatarsal joint arthrodesis. In: Functional reconstruction of the foot and ankle. Philadelphia: Lippencott Williams & Wilkins; 2000. p. 335–42.
36. Lippert FG III, McDermott JE. Crescentic osteotomy for hallux valgus: a biomechanical study of variables affecting the final position of the first metatarsal. Foot Ankle 1991;11(4):204–7.
37. Hyer CF, Glover JP, Berlet GC, et al. A comparison of the crescentic and Mau osteotomies for correction of hallux valgus. J Foot Ankle Surg 2008;47(2):103–11.
38. Trnka HJ, Hofstaetter SG, Hofstaetter JG, et al. Intermediate-term results of the Ludloff osteotomy in one hundred and eleven feet. J Bone Joint Surg Am 2008; 90(3):531–9.
39. McCluskey LC, Johnson JE, Wynarsky GT, et al. Comparison of stability of proximal crescentic metatarsal osteotomy and proximal horizontal "V" osteotomy. Foot Ankle Int 1994;15(5):263–70.
40. Markbreiter LA, Thompson FM. Proximal metatarsal osteotomy in hallux valgus correction: a comparison of crescentic and chevron procedures. Foot Ankle Int 1997;18(2):71–6.
41. Vanore JV, Christensen JC, Kravitz SR, et al. Clinical practice guideline first metatarsophalangeal joint disorders panel of the American college of foot and ankle surgeons. Diagnosis and treatment of first metatarsophalangeal joint disorders. Section 1: hallux valgus. J Foot Ankle Surg 2003;42(3):112–23.
42. Palladino SJ. Preoperative evaluation of the bunion patient. In: Gerbert J, editor. Textbook of bunion surgery. 3rd edition. Philadelphia: WB Sanders; 2001. p. 3–71.
43. Boschetti F, Pennati G, Gervaso F, et al. Biomechanical properties of human articular cartilage under compressive loads. Biorheology 2004;41(3–4):159–66.
44. Kaab MJ, Richards RG, Ito K, et al. Deformation of chondrocytes in articular cartilage under compressive load: a morphological study. Cells Tissues Organs 2003; 175(3):133–9.
45. Reverdin J. De la déviation en dehors du gros orteil (halus valgus, vulg. "oignon," "bunions," "Ballen") et de son traitement chirurgical. Transactions. International Medical Congress, 7th, London: 1881, p. 406–12 [in French].
46. Goldberg I, Bahar A, Yosipovitch Z. Late results after correction of hallux valgus deformity by basilar phalangeal osteotomy. J Bone Joint Surg Am 1987;69(1): 64–7.
47. Plattner PF, Van Manen JW. Results of Akin type proximal phalangeal osteotomy for correction of hallux valgus deformity. Orthopedics 1990;13(9):989–96.

First Metatarsophalangeal Joint Arthrodesis and Revision Arthrodesis

Graham A. Hamilton, DPM, FACFAS[a,b,]*, Lawrence A. Ford, DPM, FACFAS[b,c], Sandeep Patel, DPM[a,b]

KEYWORDS

- Hallux rigidus • Hallux valgus • Arthrodesis
- Fusion • First metatarsophalangeal joint

Disorders of the first metatarsophalangeal joint (MTPJ) are a common presenting problem to the foot and ankle surgeon. Most often, these include hallux valgus and arthritic conditions, such as hallux rigidus, posttraumatic arthritis, and rheumatoid arthritis. Each of these disorders can lead to forefoot dysfunction and have the potential for decreased load-bearing of the hallux and resultant transfer metatarsalgia. The biomechanical implications of first MTPJ arthrodesis have been well studied.[1,2] DeFrino and colleagues[1] performed a pedobarographic and gait analysis on patients after undergoing fusion of the first MTPJ. Their study demonstrated restoration of the weight-bearing function of the first ray with increased force carried through the hallux at toe-off. Brodsky's gait analysis study after first MTPJ arthrodesis revealed three major findings.[2] After fusion, patients had increased ankle push-off power, increased single limb support time, and a decrease in step width.

Hansen[3] categorized all joints of the foot and ankle as either essential or nonessential. Essential joints are those whose motion is extremely important for normal gait. Nonessential joints provide supplemental mobility. When fused they cause little or no disability with transfer stresses to the remaining joints. He defined the first MTPJ as nonessential but useful. If a first MTPJ arthrodesis is performed, little to no disability with transfer stresses to the remaining joints results. Mann[4] also noted minimal effect on patient's gait after arthrodesis. He suggested that the forefoot lifts off of the ground rapidly because of lack of the motion of the first MTPJ. This has no adverse effect on

[a] Department of Orthopedics and Podiatric Surgery, Kaiser Permanente Medical Center, 3400 Delta Fair Boulevard, Antioch, CA 94801, USA
[b] Kaiser San Francisco Bay Area Foot and Ankle Residency Program, CA, USA
[c] Department of Orthopedics and Podiatric Surgery, Kaiser Permanente Medical Center, Oakland, CA, USA
* Corresponding author.
E-mail address: graham.a.hamilton@kp.org (G.A. Hamilton).

Clin Podiatr Med Surg 26 (2009) 459–473
doi:10.1016/j.cpm.2009.03.010
0891-8422/09/$ – see front matter © 2009 Elsevier Inc. All rights reserved.

gait, and the added benefit of reducing coexisting metatarsalgia. In addition, although there is added stress on the interphalangeal joint (IPJ) with development of degenerative changes over time, this rarely becomes symptomatic.

A painful lack of motion at the first MTPJ causes a lateralization of load-bearing force during propulsion. This is explained by guarding of the symptomatic joint during push-off. Lesser metatarsal overload is often a consequence of hallux limitus.[5] Although arthroplasty of the first MTPJ can reliably eliminate pain at that joint, it does so at the expense of appropriate load-bearing. In normal feet, Stokes and coworkers[6] concluded that 30% of weight-bearing force during propulsion is carried by the hallux. The loss of intrinsic stability at the first MTPJ essentially renders the hallux and first ray useless, increasing the pressure under the central metatarsals and providing no buttress to resist overpronation of the rearfoot. Not only does arthrodesis of the first MTPJ reliably eliminate pain without compromising first ray weight-bearing, but it also has the added benefit of minimizing lateralization of forefoot loading during propulsion. The hallux must provide significant opposition to ground reactive force by increasing load-bearing of the hallux after fusion.[7]

After elimination of motion following first MTPJ arthrodesis, the lever arm of the first ray is lengthened. As the ground meets the hallux in early propulsion, the hallux in return offers resistance, and increased load. This is consistent with findings that suggest patients who underwent first MTPJ arthrodesis are more likely to return to full activities and sports than their counterparts who underwent arthroplasty.[8]

There have been numerous surgical procedures described for the treatment of hallux valgus. Similarly, arthritic conditions of the joint have been treated with cheilectomy, joint replacement, arthroplasty, decompression osteotomy, and joint fusion. This article discusses the indications and outcomes of first MTPJ arthrodesis and revision arthrodesis, their biomechanical implications, and surgical techniques.

INDICATIONS FOR FIRST METATARSOPHALANGEAL JOINT ARTHRODESIS

Arthrodesis of the first MTPJ is commonly performed for the treatment of hallux valgus and hallux rigidus. Clutton[9] first described it in 1894 for the treatment of hallux valgus. Since Clutton's original manuscript, arthrodesis has been well established as the gold standard for surgical treatment of arthritic conditions of the first MTPJ[9–12] and as a salvage procedure for failed hallux valgus surgery.[13–15] Coughlin and Shurnas[10] reviewed their long-term results of operative treatment for hallux rigidus. Thirty-four patients in their study underwent an arthrodesis procedure with a mean follow-up of 6.7 years. They reported 100% of their patients to have a good or excellent result. For patients with grade 4 and advanced grade 3 arthritis, arthrodesis was recommended. Unlike previous studies, there was no development of hallux IPJ arthrosis in this patient group. The authors reported a 94% union rate with the two asymptomatic fibrous unions.

More recently, Raikin and colleagues[16] compared outcomes of patients undergoing metallic hemiarthroplasty with those having arthrodesis for an osteoarthritic first MTPJ. With a mean follow-up of 79.4 months, their study concluded that pain score and satisfaction were significantly better in the arthrodesis group.

What is less clear in the current biomedical literature is the indication for great toe arthrodesis as a primary procedure for hallux valgus. Studies have clearly shown an excellent reduction in the intermetatarsal (IM) angle with a first MTPJ arthrodesis, without the need for proximal osteotomy.[17] Cronin and colleagues[17] performed a retrospective review of 20 patients who underwent an arthrodesis of the first MTPJ for treatment of hallux valgus. They found a mean reduction in the IM angle of 8.67 degrees (range, 5–12 degrees). The authors concluded that severe bunion deformities with degenerative changes in the joint could adequately be corrected with arthrodesis without the use of supplemental basal osteotomies. Dayton and coworkers[18] found an overall reduction of 6.41 degrees in the IM angle in their patients after surgery for moderate to severe metatarsus primus adductus. The literature has also reported favorable outcomes for the correction of hallux valgus deformity with fusion.[19] Coughlin and colleagues[19] in their retrospective review of treating moderate to severe hallux valgus with first MTPJ arthrodesis, with an average follow-up of 8 years, reported 80% of patients rated their outcome as excellent and 20% as good. There was mean IM angle correction of 6 degrees. Additional findings included complete resolution of lateral metatarsalgia. Patients had no major activity or shoe restrictions. Interestingly, 7 (33%) of the 21 patients had progressive hallux IPJ arthritis, but all changes were reported to be mild.

In a recent review, it was suggested that a grade B recommendation (supported by level III and IV evidence) could be made for the use of arthrodesis in the treatment of various hallux valgus deformities.[20]

The authors believe that first MTPJ arthrodesis provides for a predictable outcome in geriatric and rheumatoid patients with hallux valgus deformities (**Fig. 1**). It is also an excellent revisional procedure for the failed bunion with recurrent hallux valgus or iatrogenic hallux varus.[15] Finally, there should be consideration for its use in severe hallux valgus deformities with or without coexisting degenerative changes of the joint and in situations where there is a high potential for failure, such as geriatric patients with poor bone stock or spastic conditions where a strict non–weight-bearing protocol with a Lapidus arthrodesis or base osteotomy could not be tolerated (**Table 1**).

Fusion of the great toe joint is also supported by favorable union rates. A review of the literature demonstrates a nonunion rate of this procedure to be 0% to 23%.[21] The union rates have improved with advances in fixation methods and techniques in joint preparation. More recent data suggest union rates greater than 90% (**Table 2**).

TECHNIQUES
Joint Preparation

As with all fusions, joint preparation, position, and fixation are the key determinants of success. There are multiple techniques described in the literature for joint preparation. This ranges from reamers, flat cuts, curettage, and high-speed burrs.[22] The disadvantage of performing flat cuts is the technical difficulty executing the desired amount of transverse and sagittal plane correction required for optimal position. In addition, there lies an increased potential for iatrogenic shortening of the medial column leading to consequences outlined elsewhere in this issue.

Preparation of the joint surfaces is performed by curettage to maintain the contour of the joint. The ball and socket articulation allows for easy manipulation of the hallux for ideal positioning. The authors prefer using a conical reaming system for joint preparation. Once all the dorsal osteophytes are removed, a guide pin is then placed in the center of the first metatarsal head and base of the proximal phalanx and the ball and socket reamers are used to remove all joint cartilage and subchondral bone. It is important to ream without using power instrumentation, to avoid overzealous removal of bone particularly in the rheumatoid patient or patient with a poorer bone stock. Attaching the reamer to a chuck handle and controlled clockwise rotation affords excellent joint preparation. Using this technique allows for rapid joint preparation, and provides a large bone surface area for fusion. It also affords an excellent ball and socket fit with little to no gaping. There is excellent bleeding cancellous bone directly beneath the first metatarsal head, but the base of the proximal phalanx is usually more sclerotic and requires more aggressive debridement to achieve a raw bleeding surface.

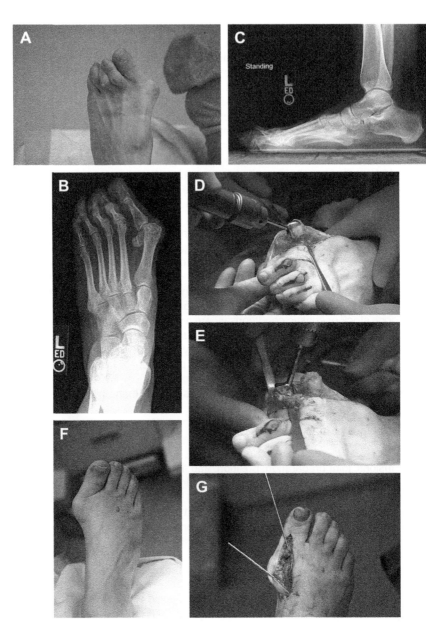

Fig. 1. (A) Clinical picture of a 67-year-old woman with chronic lesser metatarsalgia, severe hallux valgus with first ray hypermobility, and lesser digital clawtoe deformities. Patient could not tolerate a non–weight-bearing convalescence. (B, C) Anteroposterior and lateral radiographs of the patient's foot. (D, E) Clinical pictures of joint preparation using conical reamers. Note reaming is done by hand to avoid overzealous bone loss. (F, G) Clinical images of a different patient, demonstrating temporary reduction of the intermetatarsal angle with a smooth 2-mm pin before temporary fixation for the hallux. (H) Anteroposterior radiograph immediately postoperative. First MTPJ fixed with a 3.5-mm lag screw and dorsal neutralization plate. (I, J) Anteroposterior and lateral weight-bearing radiographs at 6 weeks. (K) Clinical weight-bearing image of patient at 6 weeks. (L, M) AP radiograph of a severe hallux valgus deformity. Arthrodesis achieved with crossed lag screws.

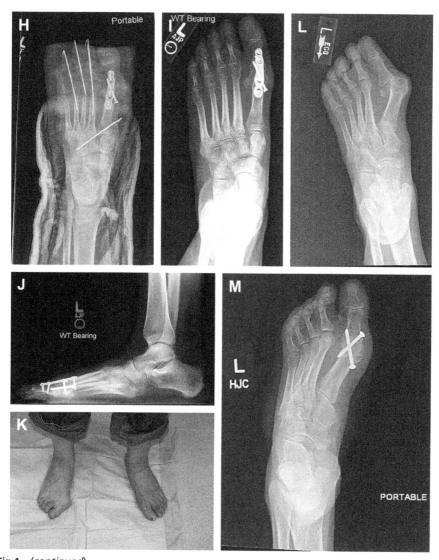

Fig. 1. (*continued*)

Position

After the joint surfaces are prepared, functional positioning is required. Alignment of the first MTPJ fusion is critical. It has been suggested that the hallux is best positioned in 10 to 15 degrees of valgus and 30 degrees of dorsiflexion relative to the first metatarsal (15 degrees to the weight-bearing surface).[8,13,23–26] These angles do not take into account the variability of foot types and function of individual patients.

The authors believe that ideal positioning should be such that, during weight-bearing, the hallux should lightly purchase the ground, parallel to the second toe in the transverse plane, and show no frontal plane deviation. This ideal weight-bearing position can be simulated intraoperatively using a number of flat surface trays. Too

Table 1	
Summary of indications for first metatarsophalangeal joint arthrodesis	
Indications	**Grafting Required**
Diffuse osteoarthritis/rheumatoid arthritis of the metatarsophalangeal joint (grade III hallux rigidus)	No
Post–avascular necrosis (bone graft needed)	Yes
Failed bunion (hallux varus or recurrent hallux valgus)	Maybe
Failed arthroplasty (Keller)	Maybe
Failed implant (bone graft needed)	Yes
Moderate to severe hallux valgus deformity	No

much dorsiflexion leads to less hallux purchase until late propulsion, which can make simple walking and shoe fitting difficult. Too much plantarflexion can lead to increased reliance on IPJ dorsiflexion, potentially increasing the rate of arthrosis at that joint. Overload of the hallux can lead to local pain or tuft callus if the joint is positioned in excessive plantarflexion. Frontal plane deviation can result in pain at the prominent condyles of the IPJ. Poor transverse plane positioning can have similar effects to an undercorrected or overcorrected hallux valgus.

Fixation

Once the corrected functional position has been obtained, and confirmed on intraoperative imaging, definitive fixation is performed. A number of methods of internal fixation have been used for this operation. These include chromic gut, K-wires, staples, specialized plates, plates, single intramedullary screw, and crossed screws.[23–25,27–32] Biomechanical cadaveric studies comparing one method of fixation with another have been conducted. Published reports are available with regard to the biomechanical strength and stiffness of different methods of fixation used in first MTPJ fusion.[23,29–32] Their clinical results, however, have not provided any definitive recommendations. For the most part joint preparation and fixation are very much surgeon dependent. Historically there has also been a trend toward higher union rates with the newer implants and techniques than the older methods.

Table 2		
Summary of nonunion rates for first metatarsophalangeal joint arthrodesis		
Author/Journal	**Fixation**	**Nonunion %**
Chana et al, JBJS, 1984	00 chromic gut/casting	10
Moynihan et al, JBJS, 1967	Wires and screws	19.4 (21 of 108)
Jardé O, Acta Orthop Belg, 2005	Screws	12 (6 of 50)
Brodsky JW, Foot Ankle Int, 2005	Screws	0 (0 of 60)
Coughlin MJ, FAI, 2005	Screws	14 (3 of 21)
Taylor DT, Am J Orthop, 2004	Screws and a dorsal plate	4 (2 of 52)
Choudhary RK, JFAS, 2004	Staples	6 (2 of 30)
Bennet GL, FAI, 2005	Screws and modular hand plate	13 (14 of 107)
Hyer CF, JFAS, 2008	Crossed screws, screws and plate	9 (4 of 45)
Sharma H, JFAS 2008	Screw, screws and dorsal plate	3 (1 of 34)

When it comes to fixation, what construct is optimal? Recently, crossed screws and specialized plates have been the mainstay of fixation for this procedure. There are extensive literature supporting favorable union rates and outcomes for these constructs.[24,29,33] The question arises for the surgeon, which construct is better? There are biomechanical studies and one clinical study that help shed light on this question. In a biomechanical study by Politi and colleagues,[33] a single screw and dorsal neutralization plate was demonstrated as being almost twice as strong as two crossed screws. Buranosky and colleagues[29] also biomechanically demonstrated that a six-hole plate with one lag screw was stiffer than two crossed lag screws.

More recently, clinical data have been published comparing screw fixation with plate constructs. Sharma and coworkers[34] compared the clinical and radiographic outcomes of patients undergoing first MTPJ fusion with a single compression screw versus a screw and one quarter tubular plate. There were no statistically significant differences between time to union, union rates, alignment, complications, and patient satisfaction. It should be noted, however, that their exclusion criteria included patients with prior history of trauma, gout, or other inflammatory or metabolic arthritides. In addition, the average body mass index was 22.2 in their patient cohort.

Similarly, Hyer and colleagues[35] looked at in vivo results comparing the use of crossed screws versus the use of a specialized plate. Again, no significant difference was found between the two groups in regards to union rates, complications, and need for hardware removal.

The results of these studies indicate that both fixation methods seem to be viable options in the low-risk patient. It is still unclear, however, whether fixation and joint preparation influence outcomes and failure rates in geriatric and high-risk bone. Further clinical studies are needed to elucidate these criteria and before definitive recommendations can be made.

Another factor to consider with fixation is the surface area of the first MTPJ. With two crossed screws surgeons often find placement of the second screw interferes with the first screw and interfragmentary compression and position can be affected. It is also intuitive that two screws crossing the joint space decrease the bone-to-bone contact. Both of these arguments support a dorsal plating technique as an easier option for fixation. Critics of a plating construct argue that patients complain of hardware problems and almost routinely require hardware removal. In the authors' experience, the rate of hardware removal of low profile and standard one third tubular plates is low. This is consistent with rate of hardware removal in the literature, which has ranged from 5% to 11%.[10,35] As well as crossed screws or a lag screw with a dorsal plate, other fixation methods have been demonstrated to be useful for first MTPJ arthrodesis.[31]

AUTHORS PREFERRED SURGICAL TECHNIQUE FOR PRIMARY ARTHRODESIS

A standard curvilinear incision is made medial to the long extensor tendon. It should extend from just proximal to the hallux IPJ crossing the MTPJ and extend approximately to about midshaft on the first metatarsal. The entire incision is usually 8 to 9 cm in length. A slightly longer incision may be necessary for easier application of the plate. If previous scars are present, then an attempt should be made to make the incision along these previous scar lines. The joint is entered through a dorsal arthrotomy and the head of the first metatarsal and base of the proximal phalanx are exposed. With severely subluxed or dislocated sesamoids, a release of the conjoint adductor tendon is also required in the first interspace. The authors have found in cases were a large IM angle is present, a percutaneous 2-mm wire can first be inserted to translate the first metatarsal laterally and reduce the IM angle. The functional position of the hallux is then assessed by loading the entire foot on a flat surface (tray cover) to simulate weight-bearing. The toe is placed in slight dorsiflexion (contacting the load-bearing surface); slight valgus (parallel with the second toe); and with no frontal plane rotation (nail plate should be parallel to the weight-bearing surface). This position is desired to simulate a functional "toe-off" position, once fusion has been attained. With the toe positioned correctly, it is temporarily stabilized with a 2-mm K-wire. Position can be checked intraoperatively using fluoroscopy or C-arm. In the anteroposterior view, the IM angle should be reduced and the sesamoids should be relocated under the first metatarsal. A congruent fit should be present at the first MTPJ with the hallux parallel with the second digit (approximately 10–15 degrees of valgus). On the lateral projection the hallux should be approximately 30 degrees to the long axis of the first metatarsal, or 10 to 15 degrees to the load-bearing surface. In some cases positioning can be challenging, such as in cases with a crossover second toe deformity or hallux valgus interphalangeus. In the case of the crossover second toe deformity, this should be addressed first and once relocated, pinned across the lesser second MTPJ so as better to assess hallux position in the transverse plane. In the case of the hallux interphalangeus, clinical position overrides radiographic position. Clinically, the hallux is positioned parallel to the second digit. Radiographically, this usually demonstrates on the anteroposterior view as a first MTPJ that is rectus (straight) or in slight varus. For these cases, such a position is optimal for fusion, as opposed to in slight valgus. If a slight valgus position is obtained patients complain of lateral hallux impingement with the second toe and callus formation.

First a cortical lag screw is placed. Here screw diameters are either 3.5 or 4 mm solid screws and usually run 28 to 40 mm in length. Many options are available as far as screw direction. It can be inserted either from the medial aspect of the first metatarsal or from the medial base of the proximal phalanx. Cannulated screws can also be used. Screw direction from the first metatarsal to the hallux is the preferred option because this causes interfragmentary compression of the fusion site with a slight valgus thrust. Directing the screw from the medial aspect of the hallux to the lateral metatarsal can cause the toe to shift into a slight varus alignment as the screw is tightened. Once the first lag screw is placed, either a second lag screw is used or a dorsal neutralization plate is contoured to the dorsal surface of the first metatarsal and proximal phalanx. In the latter, a standard one third tubular plate can be used ensuring at least four cortices are engaged with compression screws proximal and distal to the joint line.

In the patient with more porotic bone, a locking fixed-angle plate can be used. There are also many commercially available low-profile precontoured fixed-angle specialty plates. These can be beneficial in the patient with poorer bone stock, but they are not required in all cases.

POSTOPERATIVELY

With the advent of newer implants, patients have the ability to ambulate on the foot almost immediately after surgery. The authors' protocol is a short leg-walking cast for 6 weeks and then a surgical shoe or tennis shoe.

Dayton and McCall[36] walked all 18 patients immediately after fusion in a postoperative shoe. Union was achieved on average in 6.1 weeks and patients were on average in an athletic shoe at 6.23 weeks. Hyer and coworkers[35] reported similar findings in 37 patients who were allowed to bear weight immediately, with a fusion rate of 91.1%.

REVISION ARTHRODESIS

A challenging problem surgeons confront is how surgically to manage cases of first MTPJ nonunion, malunion, and failed implant or Keller arthroplasty. Patients with this problem usually present complaining of pain, deformity, or both at the first MTPJ, or the lesser metatarsophalangeal joints. The cause of the pain or deformity can be multifactorial, from chronic synovitis and swelling around the hardware and pseudoarthrosis, to hardware breakage, to biomechanical disruption of first ray stability and resultant lesser metatarsophalangeal joint overload.

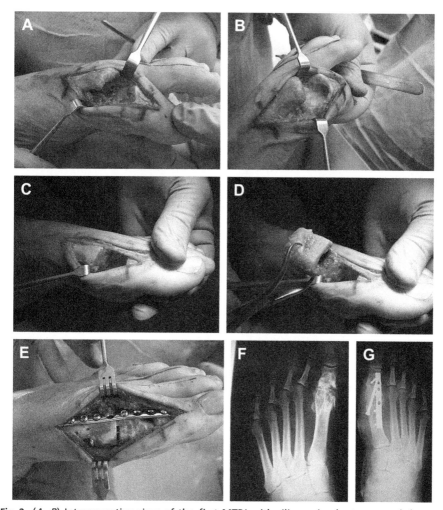

Fig. 2. (*A*, *B*) Intraoperative view of the first MTPJ with silicone implant removed demonstrating erosion of the proximal phalanx and first metatarsal head. (*C*) Autogenous cancellous bone graft with demineralized bone matrix packing the "defects." (*D*, *E*) Intraoperative views demonstrating structural tricortical iliac crest graft. Graft in place with internal fixation. (*F*) Anteroposterior radiograph of a symptomatic failed Silastic implant with varus subluxation of the hallux second and third digits. Extensive preoperative cystic change of the proximal phalanx and first metatarsal head is evident. (*G*) Anteroposterior radiograph of a first MTPJ distraction arthrodesis.

Despite the reported failures associated with first MTPJ arthrodesis, there is a paucity of literature on how to salvage these failures. Salvage can be particularly difficult in the younger, active patient. Options include living with the pain, conversion to a Keller arthroplasty, or bone block distraction arthrodesis.

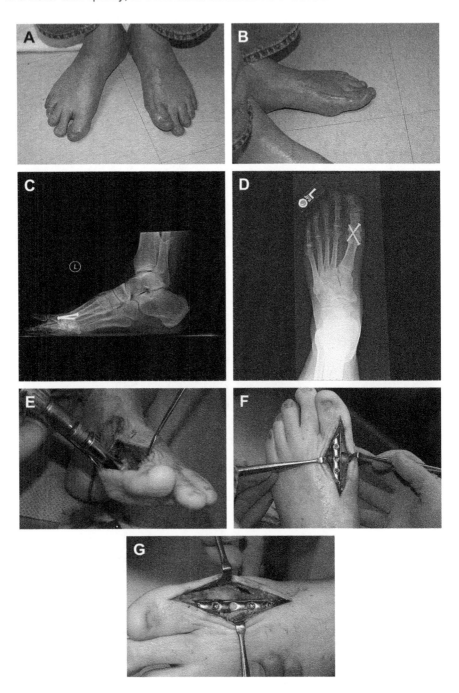

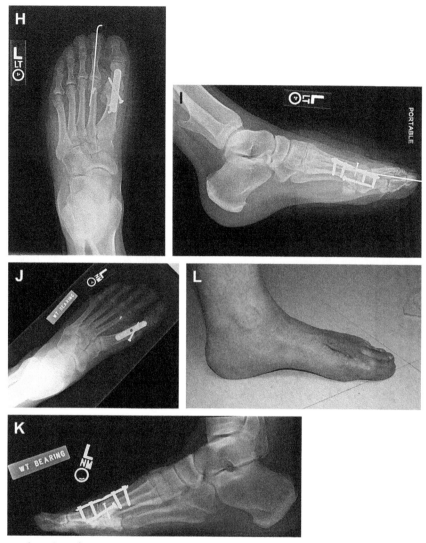

Fig. 3. (*continued*)

Fig. 3. (*A, B*) Clinical picture of a patient with previous first MTPJ arthrodesis and malunion. Patient complained of inadequate toe purchase, shoeing, and pain under the second MTPJ. (*C, D*) Preoperative weight-bearing AP and lateral projections demonstrating dorsiflexion malunion of the first MTPJ. (*E*) Osteotomy performed of the first MTPJ using a crescentic blade. The blade was passed from medial to lateral to facilitate sagittal plane correction. (*F, G*) Fixation with a lag screw and dorsal one third tubular locking plate. (*H, I, J*) Postoperative AP and lateral radiographs. A Weil osteotomy of the second metatarsal and PIPJ arthrodesis of the second toe was also performed. (*J, K, L*) Six weeks postoperative radiographs with solid union and a plantigrade hallux. (*L*) Clinical image of foot showing good toe position and purchase.

For the older more sedentary individual with low physical demands, hardware removal with conversion to a Keller resectional arthroplasty is an option. It must be remembered that this option does not provide a functional forefoot even for the minimally active patient. Patients must be counseled on the strong possibility of lesser metatarsal overload symptoms and the need for orthoses postoperatively. Many authors have reported postoperative lesser metatarsalgia in active patients after resectional arthroplasty of the first MTPJ.[37,38]

Revision bone-block arthrodesis is the procedure of choice for the medically fit, active individual with a failed fusion. It is the most biomechanically sound option and, if successful, accomplishes several goals. Subjectively, it improves patient's levels of pain and walking tolerance. Objectively, it restores first ray stability alleviating lesser MTPJ overload symptoms. It also affords restoration of great toe alignment and length and once hallux position is restored lesser digital malalignment can be corrected. Hecht and colleagues[39] looked at functional outcomes of distraction arthrodesis after a failed implant in a series of 14 patients. They reported an 80% union rate and 20% nonunion rate. The authors stipulated that this procedure, although technically demanding, provides long-term stability to the hallux, restores weight-bearing, and allows for maintenance of a propulsive gait. Brodsky and coworkers[40] reported on first MTPJ salvage with ipsilateral calcaneal bone graft (ICBG). Eight were from failed implants, two from avascular necrosis, one a nonunion, and one with chronic osteomyelitis. The union rate was 92%. The major disadvantage is risk of nonunion. Fusion must occur at two interfaces at a location in the foot that relies on relatively small vessels providing perfusion.

Pre-operative Planning

Preoperative anteroposterior, lateral, and medial oblique weight-bearing radiographs of both feet should be obtained before surgery. This allows for assessment of the "good foot" to compare and contrast digital malalignment, shortening, and bony erosion about the hardware. It also allows the surgeon the ability to assess the metatarsal parabola. Patients should be counseled of the need for autogenous bone graft and of the risk of further morbidity from the bone graft donor site. Usually, three donor sites are potentially used depending on the size of the graft needed. If a 1 to 1.5 cm in length piece is required then a bicortical block of bone can be harvested from the superior aspect of the calcaneus or distal tibia. If a larger piece is needed, then a tricortical bone block from the anterior iliac crest is the best option. Preoperative radiographs give the surgeon an idea of the size of structural graft needed. Demineralized bone matrix and other osteogenic products can be mixed with autogenous cancellous bone to "fill" defects created by the implant. Rigid fixation is required until union is obtained. Fixation is usually internal, but external fixators can be used to add to the construct.

Authors Preferred Surgical Technique

The patient is positioned supine and the foot and ipsilateral hip are prepared and draped. If the heel is the site for bone harvesting, then a bump is placed under the hip. If possible the incision over the first MTPJ is made over any existing scars. The dorsal linear incision usually measures 8 to 9 cm in length and is placed just medial to the long extensor tendon. The incision is carried to bone and the joint is entered. All implants are removed and fibrous tissue debrided. The bone interfaces are resected with an oscillating saw and high-speed burr until bleeding is noted. Once the fibrous margins have been removed, the defects can be packed with cancellous bone and orthobiologics to promote osteogenesis. The structural graft is then fashioned to fit the defect, restoring a plantigrade hallux with good length. Often with these cases, a varus malposition is observed of the hallux and second and third digits. These digits can usually be anatomically aligned once the hallux is anatomically positioned. With the graft in place and of appropriate length, it is fixed with an obliquely placed 3.5- or 4-mm AO positional cortex screw and a five- to seven-hole one third tubular dorsal neutralization plate. The positional screw length usually measures 40 to 60 mm in length and is directed from the medial aspect of the first metatarsal head through the graft, to the lateral aspect of the base of the proximal phalanx. The plate is positioned slightly lateral to midline of the metatarsal and hallux for coverage with the extensor tendon. At least four cortices should be engaged both proximal and distal the graft piece. Sometimes given the extent of sclerosis in the proximal phalanx, this is not always achievable because the residual proximal phalanx after resection can be extremely short. In such cases a fixed-angle plate is preferable. The extensor tendon is reapproximated over the plate and the remaining layers are closed (**Fig. 2**). Postoperatively, patients are placed into a modified Jones compression splint for 10 to 14 days, at which time sutures are removed. A short-leg non–weight-bearing cast is applied for 4 more weeks. Non–weight-bearing radiographs of the foot are taken when the patient returns for follow-up examination at 6 weeks postoperatively. Depending on radiographic healing, patients are advanced to a removable, fiberglass walking boot, and partial weight-bearing for 2 weeks followed by full weight-bearing for another 2 weeks in the walking boot. Evidence of radiographic consolidation determines advancement to regular supportive shoes and regular activities as tolerated. Follow-up visits and weight-bearing radiographs of the foot are repeated at 3 and 6 months postoperatively. Given the higher risk of delayed union or nonunion, external bone stimulation is also routinely recommended for these cases, particularly if the structural graft piece exceeds 2 cm in length.

In the case of malunion the authors have found alignment can be restored with a crescentic osteotomy. This recreates a ball and socket joint, which can then be fixed with a screw and plate construct once the great toe has been realigned (**Fig. 3**).

SUMMARY

First MTPJ arthrodesis has clearly been established as the gold standard for the treatment of end-stage hallux rigidus. It also provides for a predictable and reproducible outcome in geriatric and rheumatoid patients with symptomatic hallux valgus. The procedure should also be considered for the patient with severe hallux valgus with or without coexisting degenerative changes of the joint, where a strict non–weight-bearing protocol with a Lapidus arthrodesis or base osteotomy could not be tolerated. First MTPJ is also an excellent revision procedure for the failed bunion with recurrent hallux valgus or iatrogenic hallux varus.

Biomechanically, first MTPJ arthrodesis causes little to no disability with transfer stresses to the remaining joints and has little adverse effect on gait. Arthrodesis of the first MTPJ also restores the weight-bearing function of the first ray with increased force carried through the hallux at toe-off. With the weight-bearing function of the first ray restored, this in turn reduces the risk of transfer metatarsalgia.

Revision bone-block arthrodesis is the procedure of choice for the medically fit, active individual with a failed fusion. It is the most biomechanically sound option and if successful, it accomplishes several goals. Subjectively, it improves the patient's levels of pain and walking tolerance. Objectively, it restores first ray stability alleviating lesser MTPJ overload symptoms. It also affords restoration of great toe alignment and length and once hallux position is restored lesser digital malalignment can be corrected.

REFERENCES

1. DeFrino PF, Brodsky JW, Pollo FE, et al. First metatarsophalangeal arthrodesis: a clinical, pedobarographic and gait analysis study. Foot Ankle Int 2002;23(6): 496–502.
2. Brodsky JW, Baum BS, Pollo FE, et al. Prospective gait analysis in patients with first metatarsophalangeal joint arthrodesis for hallux rigidus. Foot Ankle Int 2007;28(2):162–5.
3. Hansen ST Jr. Functional reconstruction of the foot and ankle. Pennsylvania: Lippincott and Williams; 2000. p. 30–2.
4. Mann RA. Surgical implications of biomechanics of the foot and ankle. Clin Orthop Relat Res 1980;146:111–8.
5. Beertema W, Draijer WF, van Os JJ, et al. A retrospective analysis of surgical treatment in patients with symptomatic hallux rigidus: long-term follow-up. J Foot Ankle Surg 2006;45(4):244–51.
6. Stokes IAF, Hutton WC, Stott JRR. Forces acting on the metatarsals during normal walking. J Anat 1979;129(3):579–90.
7. Budhabhatti SP, Erdemir A, Petre M, et al. Finite element modeling of the first ray of the foot: a tool for the design of interventions. J Biomech Eng 2007;129(5): 750–6.
8. Bouché RT, Adad JM. Arthrodesis of the first metatarsophalangeal joint in active people. Clin Podiatr Med Surg 1996;13(3):461–84.
9. Clutton HH. The treatment of hallux valgus. St Thomas Rep 1894;22:1–12.
10. Coughlin MJ, Shurnas PS. Hallux rigidus: grading and long-term results of operative treatment. J Bone Joint Surg Am 2003;85(11):2072–88.
11. Shereff MJ, Baumhauer JF. Hallux rigidus and osteoarthrosis of the first metatarsophalangeal joint. J Bone Joint Surg Am 1998;80(6):898–908.
12. Lombardi CM, Silhanek AD, Connolly FG, et al. First metatarsophalangeal arthrodesis for treatment of hallux rigidus: a retrospective study. J Foot Ankle Surg 2001;40(3):137–43.
13. Wu KK. First metatarsophalangeal fusion in the salvage of failed hallux abducto valgus operations. J Foot Ankle Surg 1994;33(4):383–95.
14. Vienne P, Sukthankar A, Favre P, et al. Metatarsophalangeal joint arthrodesis after failed Keller-Brandes procedure. Foot Ankle Int 2006;27(11):894–901.
15. Grimes JS, Coughlin MJ. First metatarsophalangeal joint arthrodesis as a treatment for failed hallux valgus surgery. Foot Ankle Int 2006;27(11):887–93.
16. Raikin SM, Ahmad J, Pour AE, et al. Comparison of arthrodesis and metallic hemiarthroplasty of the hallux metatarsophalangeal joint. J Bone Joint Surg Am 2007; 89(9):1979–85.
17. Cronin JJ, Limbers JP, Kutty S, et al. Intermetatarsal angle after first metatarsophalangeal joint arthrodesis for hallux valgus. Foot Ankle Int 2006;27(2):104–9.
18. Dayton P, LoPiccolo J, Kiley J. Reduction of the intermetatarsal angle after first metatarsophalangeal joint arthrodesis in patients with moderate to severe metatarsus primus adductus. J Foot Ankle Surg 2002;41:316–9.
19. Coughlin MJ, Grebing BR, Jones CP. Arthrodesis of the first metatarsophalangeal joint for idiopathic hallux valgus: intermediate results. Foot Ankle Int 2005;26(10): 783–92.
20. Easley ME, Trnka H. Current concepts review: hallux valgus part II: operative treatment. Foot Ankle Int 2007;6:748–58.
21. Gimple K, Anspacher JC, Kopta JA. Metatarsophalangeal joint fusion of the great toe. Orthopaedics 1978;1:462–7.

22. Johansson JE, Barrington TW. Cone arthrodesis of the first metatarsophalangeal joint. Foot Ankle 1984;4:244–8.
23. Curtis MJ, Myerson M, Jinnah RH, et al. Arthrodesis of the first metatarsophalangeal joint: a biomechanical study of internal fixation techniques. Foot Ankle 1993; 14(7):395–9.
24. Coughlin MJ, Abdo RV. Arthrodesis of first metatarsophalangeal joint with Vitallium plate fixation. Foot Ankle 1994;15:18–28.
25. Riggs SA, Johnson EW, McKeever D. Arthrodesis for the painful hallux. Foot Ankle 1983;3:248–53.
26. Fitzgerald JA, Wilkinson JM. Arthrodesis of the metatarsophalangeal joint of the great toe. Clin Orthop Relat Res 1981;157:70–7.
27. O'Doherty DP, Lowrie IG, Magnussen PA, et al. The management of painful first metatarsophalangeal joint in the older patient: arthrodesis or Keller arthroplasty? J Bone Joint Surg Br 1990;72:839–42.
28. Watson AD, Kelikian AS. Cost effectiveness comparison of three methods of internal fixation for arthrodesis of the first metatarsophalangeal joint. Foot Ankle Int 1988;19(5):304–10.
29. Buranosky DJ, Taylor DT, Sage RA, et al. First metatarsophalangeal joint arthrodesis: quantitative mechanical testing of six hole dorsal plate versus crossed screw fixation in cadaveric specimens. J Foot Ankle Surg 2001;40(4):208–13.
30. Molloy S, Burkhart BG, Jasper BS, et al. Biomechanical comparison of two fixation methods for first metatarsophalangeal joint arthrodesis. Foot Ankle Int 2001;24(2):169–71.
31. Neufeld SK, Parks BG, Naseef GS, et al. Arthrodesis of the first metatarsophalangeal joint: a biomechanical study comparing memory compression staples, cannulated screws, and a dorsal plate. Foot Ankle Int 2002;23(2):97–101.
32. Sage RA, Lam AT, Taylor DT. Retrospective analysis of first metatarsophalangeal joint arthrodesis. J Foot Ankle Surg 1997;36:425–9.
33. Politi J, John H, Njus G, et al. First metatarsal-phalangeal joint arthrodesis: a biomechanical assessment of stability. Foot Ankle Int 2003 Apr;24(4):332–7.
34. Sharma H, Bhagat S, Deleeuw J, et al. In vivo comparison of screw versus plate and screw fixation for first metatarsophalangeal arthrodesis: does augmentation of internal compression screw fixation using a semi-tubular plate shorten time to clinical and radiologic fusion of the first metatarsophalangeal joint (MTPJ)? J Foot Ankle Surg 2008;47(1):2–7.
35. Hyer CF, Glover JP, Berlet GC, et al. Cost comparison of crossed screws versus dorsal plate construct for first metatarsophalangeal joint arthrodesis. J Foot Ankle Surg 2008;47(1):13–8.
36. Dayton P, McCall A. Early weightbearing after first metatarsophalangeal joint arthrodesis: a retrospective observational case analysis. J Foot Ankle Surg 2004;43(3):156–9.
37. Bonney G, MacNab L. Hallux valgus and hallux rigidus: a critical survey of operative results. J Bone Joint Surg Br 1952;34:366–85.
38. Cleveland M, Winant EM. An end-result of the Keller operation. J Bone Joint Surg Am 1950;32:163–75.
39. Hecht PJ, Gibbons MJ, Wapner KL, et al. Arthrodesis of the first metatarsophalangeal joint to salvage failed silicone implant arthroplasty. Foot Ankle Int 1997;18(7): 383–90.
40. Brodsky JW, Ptaszek AJ, Morris SG. Salvage first MTP arthrodesis utilizing ICBG: clinical evaluation and outcome. Foot Ankle Int 2000;21(4):290–6.

Complications and Revisional Hallux Valgus Surgery

Ronald Belczyk, DPM[a], John J. Stapleton, DPM[b,c],
Jordan P. Grossman, DPM, FACFAS[d], Thomas Zgonis, DPM, FACFAS[a,*]

KEYWORDS

- Revisional surgery • Hallux valgus • Hallux varus
- Bunion • Complications

The rate of complications following hallux valgus surgery is variable and has been reported as ranging from 1% to 55% in the scientific literature.[1–10] Questions about the reasons for failed hallux valgus surgery become even more difficult when one considers individual patient needs and expectations. Although it is important to choose the appropriate procedure on the basis of a number of factors including clinical and radiographic presentation, it is equally important to offer the appropriate treatment recommendations based on the patient's past medical history and ability to comply with postoperative recommendations and in accord with his or her lifestyle.

When the surgeon fails to recognize these issues and to discuss them preoperatively, it becomes much more difficult to manage the patient's care postoperatively should a complication arise. Before making any treatment recommendation for revisional hallux valgus correction, one may need to review all pertinent medical records, including the patient's history and physical examinations, progress notes, operative reports, and all radiographs, to understand the cause of surgical failure.

Although the rate of complications varies from investigator to investigator, it ultimately depends on the surgeon's expertise in patient and procedural selection, ability to perform the surgery selected, and knowledge in dealing with perioperative issues and complications. The complications are numerous and not limited to those listed in **Box 1**. Some of the most common complications encountered include recurrent hallux valgus, hallux varus, malunion, and avascular necrosis (AVN).

[a] Division of Podiatric Medicine and Surgery, Department of Orthopaedic Surgery, The University of Texas Health Science Center at San Antonio, 7703 Floyd Curl Drive, San Antonio, TX 78229, USA
[b] Foot and Ankle Surgery, VSAS Orthopaedics, 1250 S Cedar Street, Allentown, PA 18103, USA
[c] Penn State College of Medicine, 500 University Drive, Hershey, PA 17033, USA
[d] Department of Surgery, Saint Vincent Charity Hospital, 2351 East 22nd Street, Cleveland, OH 44115, USA
* Corresponding author.
E-mail address: zgonis@uthscsa.edu (T. Zgonis).

Clin Podiatr Med Surg 26 (2009) 475–484
doi:10.1016/j.cpm.2009.04.002
0891-8422/09/$ – see front matter © 2009 Elsevier Inc. All rights reserved.

podiatric.theclinics.com

Box 1
Potential complications reported following hallux valgus surgery

- Avascular necrosis
- Fracture
- Hallux extensus
- Hallux varus
- Hematoma
- Inadequate correction or recurrent hallux valgus
- Incisional neuroma
- Soft tissue infection
- Osteomyelitis
- Lack of propulsion
- Malunion
- Nonunion
- Stiffness
- Suture reaction
- Toe shortening
- Transfer metatarsalgia

RECURRENT HALLUX VALGUS

Numerous operations have been described for the correction of hallux valgus deformities. Most reported operations have satisfactory clinical results, but each has associated risks of complications and failures. Notably, the incidence of recurrence following hallux valgus surgery has been reported to be as high as 16%.[10] Asymptomatic recurrences can be treated with observation and nonoperative intervention; however, when symptoms persist and revisional surgery becomes an option, further work-up is needed to determine the cause for recurrence (**Box 2**).

There are several considerations with revisional cases, and it is helpful to obtain presurgical radiographs to determine whether the recurrent hallux valgus deformity is secondary to improper procedural selection. The location of the osteotomy is often dictated by the amount of correction needed.[8] In addition to clinical evaluation, the typical radiographic parameters used to determine the most appropriate procedure include the intermetatarsal (IM) angle, hallux valgus angle, distal metatarsal articular angle, position of the sesamoids, length of the first ray, shape of the cuneiform, and joint incongruity of the first metatarsophalangeal joint (MTPJ) and first metatarsocuneiform joint (MCJ). Despite the reliability of inter-/intraobserver radiographic measurements, choosing an inadequate procedure can lead to undercorrection or recurrence. For instance, selecting a distal metatarsal osteotomy (DMO) for a severe hallux valgus deformity results in recurrence. The amount of lateral translation possible with a DMO is limited by the width of the metatarsal, and achieving fixation of the osteotomy becomes more difficult when the capital fragment is translated more than 50%. Another potential source of error occurs with a lowered estimation of the IM angle in the metatarsus adductus foot type. The true IM angle in this foot type accounts for the measured IM angle plus the amount of increased metatarsus adductus angle.

Box 2
Potential causes for recurrent hallux valgus deformity

- Inadequate lateral release
- Inadequate intermetatarsal correction
- Lack of medial capsular repair
- Improper procedural selection
- Not addressing valgus deformity at the interphalangeal joint
- Not addressing hindfoot abnormality
- Underestimation of intermetatarsal angle by not considering a metatarsus adductus deformity
- Metatarsocuneiform joint instability
- Inadequate fixation or mechanical failure of hardware
- Patient noncompliance

In addition, underlying sagittal or transverse plane instability of the first MCJ may not have been recognized preoperatively and can be a source of recurrent deformity. Although basal osteotomies of the first metatarsal have been reported to decrease the mobility of the tarsometatarsal (TMT) joints, this does not occur following DMO. With revisional cases, it is important to evaluate motion at the first TMT, digital contractures, plantar callosities, plantar gapping at the first TMT on a lateral radiograph, cortical hypertrophy of the second metatarsal, increased IM angle, and the presence of generalized ligamentous laxity—all of which may suggest hypermobility (see **Box 2**).

Consideration should also be given to the integrity of the surrounding soft tissue apparatus and its dynamic stabilization about the first MTPJ. Inadequate reconstruction or persistent laxity of the medial capsule can be a potential source of deformity. Transection or laxity of the medial capsule significantly destabilizes the first MTPJ, leading to hallux valgus deformity, thus implying that operative correction should entail some form of medial capsular repair. The numerous ways of repairing the medial capsule are not reported in all cases for hallux valgus correction.

Several surgical options exist for the management of a recurrent hallux valgus deformity: first metatarsal osteotomies, resection arthroplasty, first MTPJ fusion, and first MCJ fusion. These osseous procedures have to be combined with capsulotendinous soft tissue balancing to achieve correction. The resection arthroplasty removes the proximal third of the first proximal phalanx and is occasionally combined with a distal soft tissue procedure such as fibular sesamoidectomy, medial capsulorraphy, extensor tendon lengthening, tendon transfer, or Z skin plasty. Resection arthroplasty has been historically reserved for elderly patients who have limited functional demands due to potential complications of transfer metatarsalgia, shortening of the hallux, and loss of hallux purchase. The modified Lapidus has been described as a salvage procedure after failed surgical treatment of hallux valgus deformity.[1] Although the originally described Lapidus was an arthrodesis between the bases of the first and second metatarsals and the first intercuneiform joint, the modified Lapidus procedure incorporates an isolated arthrodesis of the first TMT joint with a lateral and plantar-based closing wedge osteotomy of the medial cuneiform. The arthrodesis can also be performed by maintaining the contour of the joint and by using the shape of the joint to achieve the necessary correction. The main advantage of this technique is that further shortening of the osteotomy is avoided. Although there is controversy regarding the presence of hypermobility with hallux valgus deformities, the modified Lapidus eliminates any transverse and sagittal hypermobility that may exist with revisional cases. Lastly, first MTPJ fusion has been successfully used as an isolated procedure for severe hallux valgus deformities when there is a large IM angle or when there is MTPJ arthrosis or stiffness.[3] In addition, various proximal osteotomies can be used to correct residual deformity, because they have been shown to achieve significant correction of the IM angle (**Figs. 1** and **2**).

HALLUX VARUS

Hallux varus is an abnormal medial deviation of the hallux following overcorrection of a hallux valgus deformity. Contemporary shoe gear, commonly tapered at the toe box, makes even mild varus deformities difficult and painful. Other patients present because of the cosmetic disfigurement of the toe and foot. The usual symptoms encountered with hallux varus include deformity, pain, decreased range of motion, and developing arthrosis of the first MTPJ instability about the first MPTJ, clawing of the first toe, weakness with push-off, and shoewear problems. It can present as

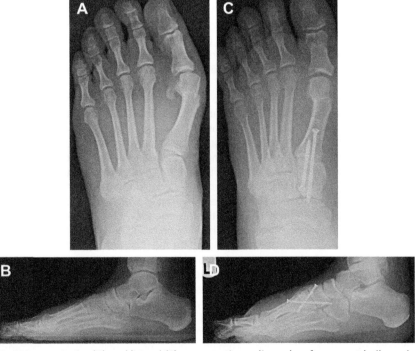

Fig. 1. Anteroposterior (A) and lateral (B) preoperative radiogaphs of recurrent hallux valgus after a distal first metatarsal osteotomy was performed for a severe deformity. This procedure selection was obviously inappropriate for this particular deformity. Postoperative anteroposterior (C) and lateral radiographs (D) after realignment with a first MCJ arthrodesis to correct all components of recurrent deformity and stabilize the first ray/medial column. Note realignment of the first ray in the sagittal and transverse planes and anatomic position of the first MTPJ.

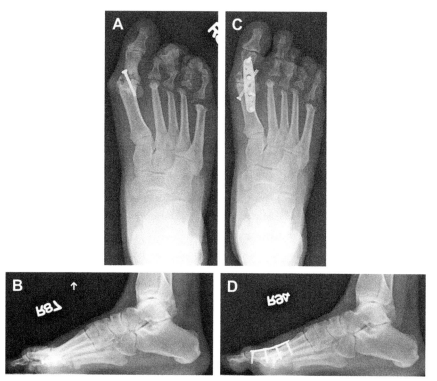

Fig. 2. Anteroposterior (*A*) and lateral (*B*) preoperative radiographs of a recurrent hallux valgus deformity after a nonunion of the first MTPJ. Patient also had resection of the lesser metatarsal heads and complained of pain to the first and second digits. Postoperative anteroposterior (*C*) and lateral radiographs (*D*) after realignment with a revisional first MTPJ arthrodesis and second-digit arthrodesis at the proximal interphalangeal joint.

early as the time of intraoperative correction or can be a progressive deformity that presents months later secondary to a muscular imbalance about the first MTPJ.

Box 3 lists the potential causes for this deformity present in revision cases. Hallux varus can result from a number of causes including and not limited to poor capsular repair or tissue handling, poor selection of operative procedure (eg, a soft tissue procedure for a functionally adapted joint), lengthening of the first ray by way of lengthening osteotomy, dorsiflexion malunion, poor surgical planning, failing to consider functional hallux limitus preoperatively, excessive shortening of the abductor hallucis muscle, excessive resection of the medial eminence, removal of the fibular sesamoid, excessive correction of the first IM angle, overaggressive postoperative dressing application, aggressive lateral release including the conjoined tendon of the adductor with the lateral capsule and lateral flexor hallucis brevis, iatrogenic tendon tear, prolonged first metatarsal phalangeal immobilization, and poor patient compliance.

Preoperatively, one needs to assess the reducibility of the of the hallux varus deformity or contracture at the interphalangeal joint, stiffness of the MTPJ, pain with range of motion at the MTPJ, and the strength of the flexor hallucis longus or extensor hallucis longus tendons. Preoperative template planning can also help identify other forefoot or hindfoot abnormalities and plan the location and degree of angular correction needed at the metatatarsal or phalanx. In many cases, iatrogenic-caused hallux varus

---

Box 3
Potential causes for hallux varus deformity following hallux valgus surgery

- Aggressive lateral release including the conjoined tendon of the adductor with the lateral capsule and lateral flexor hallucis brevis
- Dorsiflexion malunion
- Excessive shortening of the abductor hallucis muscle
- Excessive resection of the medial eminence
- Excision of the fibular sesamoid
- Excessive correction of the 1–2 IM angle
- Iatrogenic tendon tear
- Lengthening of the first ray by way of lengthening osteotomy
- Overaggressive medial capsule plication
- Overaggressive postoperative dressing application
- Poor surgical planning; failing to consider functional hallux limitus preoperatively
- Poor capsular repair or tissue handling
- Poor selection of operative procedure (eg, a soft tissue procedure for a functionally adapted joint)
- Prolonged first metatarsal phalangeal immobilization
- Poor patient compliance

---

can be prevented at the time of surgery. For instance, the surgeon can avoid excessive resection of the medial eminence by performing this procedure following IM angle correction from a proximal metatarsal osteotomy or metatarsal cuneiform arthrodesis. A simple bunionectomy that involves overzealous resection of the dorsal medial eminence and violation of the sagittal groove can potentially lead to dislocation of the tibial sesamoid and medial soft tissue contractures. A hallux varus deformity can also occur from an aggressive soft tissue lateral release. When the adductor hallucis, the lateral head of the flexor hallucis brevis, and the lateral capsule of the MTPJ are all released, there is no opposition to the medial soft tissue structures. Even when the lateral capsule is left intact, it is often unable to resist the medial forces of the abductor hallucis, the medial head of the flexor hallucis brevis, and the extensor hallucis longus. In summary, surgeons should avoid overcorrection of the IM angle and be aware of the potential complications of an aggressive lateral release or medial capsule repair.

Some surgeons may believe that mild asymptomatic hallux varus deformities should be treated nonoperatively with extradepth shoewear. The dilemma arises as when to operate on a hallux varus deformity. Often, the surgeon cannot assume that the hallux varus that is asymptomatic initially will not become symptomatic. In addition, the progression of arthrosis and associated joint stiffness as a result of the hallux varus must be considered because it is likely to occur. For these reasons, surgeons have a low threshold for revisional surgery when a hallux varus deformity is encountered. Numerous procedures have been described by various investigators for the correction of the reducible nonarthritic hallux varus deformity. Some of these soft tissue procedures include lengthening of the abductor hallucis, plication of the lateral capsule, extensor brevis tenodesis, and a reverse transfer of the abductor hallucis tendon (**Table 1**). The purpose of the abductor transfer procedure is to stabilize the lateral

Table 1	
Soft tissue procedures for correction of hallux varus	
Procedure	Rationale
Lengthening of the abductor hallucis	Corrects contracture of the abductor hallucis
Medial capsulotomy	Releases medial soft tissue contracture
Lateral capsule repair	Tightens up the lateral capsule to the MPJ
Repair of the conjoined tendon to the adductor hallucis	Repairs the transected tendon
Extensor hallucis longus tendon transfer	
Split extensor hallucis longus tendon transfer	
Free tendon grafts	
Extensor hallucis brevis tenodesis	Provides static restraint for flexible deformity
A reverse transfer of the abductor hallucis tendon	Static stabilization of the lateral soft tissue complex

soft tissue components of the first MTPJ.[9] Soft tissue procedures may be useful for mild cases, but the surgeon should not rely on soft tissue procedures to compensate for osseous deformities. For example, an overcorrected IM angle has to be corrected with a revisional osteotomy or arthrodesis to adequately correct the deformity because soft tissue procedures may seem sufficient initially but will ultimately fail (**Fig. 3**).

When soft tissue and osseous adaptation develop, it makes joint salvage procedures more difficult. In general, tendon transfers potentially avoid the limitations associated with fusion; however, when the deformity is severe (not reducible, stiff, or painful), resection or arthrodesis of the MTPJ is recommended as a salvage procedure (**Table 2**).[2,4,6,7]

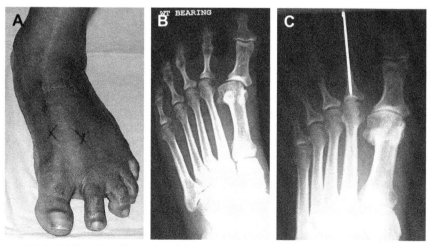

Fig. 3. Clinical (*A*) and radiographic (*B*) preoperative views of an iatrogenic hallux varus deformity. (*C*) Postoperative view after correction of the hallux varus deformity with soft tissue balancing procedures. Note that a second-digit arthrodesis was also performed. WT, weight.

Table 2	
Osseous procedures for correction of hallux varus	
Procedure	Rationale
Ostetotomy	Increases the IM angle
Hallux interphalangeal joint (IPJ) arthrodesis	Corrects the deformity at the IPJ and used in conjunction with extensor hallucis longus tendon transfer
Bone grafting to the medial side of the first MTPJ	Restores the bone loss from aggressive medial eminence resection
First MTPJ arthrodesis	Permanent reduction and stabilization of the first MTPJ position

Arthrodesis is a versatile procedure that can be performed following failed proximal and distal osteotomies, arthrodesis of the MCJ, McBride procedure, exostectomy, and resection arthroplasty.[4] Static and dynamic influences on the first MTPJ are unpredictable following failed hallux valgus correction, and the authors prefer an arthrodesis procedure as a method of permanently reducing and stabilizing the first MTPJ.

MALUNION

Malunion of the first metatarsal is a poorly tolerated complication. Dorsal angulation and metarsus primus elevatus can lead to transfer metatarsalgia or callosities and pain of the first MTPJ. It is important to recognize this intraoperatively at the time of hallux valgus correction or immediately after surgery. With early recognition, it is easy to return the patient to the operating room, correct the malunion, and add greater skeletal stability.

Malunions may occur due to improper intraoperative position, failure of fixation, performing an unstable osteotomy with inappropriate fixation, and patient noncompliance. A failure to maintain adequate position following an osteotomy depends on the stability of the osteotomy and the method of fixation. Greater stability is afforded with V-shaped osteotomies compared with opening/closing osteotomies that require an intact cortex for stability. The type of fixation should be appropriate for the quality of bone, the location and design of the osteotomy, and the patient's ability to comply with postoperative recommendations. Due to various potential intraoperative challenges such as fractures sustained intraoperatively from osteotomy or placement of internal fixation, osteopenia, or poor purchase of screws, the stability of fixation should be assessed intraoperatively. The surgeon needs to be capable of various methods of fixation should the primary approach fail. Proximal osteotomies are subjected to particularly high stresses; the complication rate of dorsal angulation has been reported to be as high as 82% for certain procedures.[11-18]

The treatment of malunions often requires osteotomy of the first metatarsal to correct the osseous component of the deformity. The purpose of such osteotomy procedures is to normalize the alignment of the first ray to restore its function during gait.

AVASCULAR NECROSIS

AVN of the first metatarsal is uncommon; however, it has been reported to occur following hallux valgus correction with distal metatarsal osteotomies. The incidence of AVN is variable following distal chevron osteotomy.[5,11,12,14,16] The potential causes for AVN are many and include local and systemic factors.

Local factors include (but are not limited to) thermal necrosis from the use of power instrumentation and excessive dissection around the first MTPJ. Locally, the arterial network entering the dorsolateral aspect of the first metatarsal is at risk by violation of the lateral cortex of the first metatarsal at the time of the osteotomy. The extraosseous blood supply to the metatarsal head will also be seriously damaged if the dorsal, lateral, or inferior capsular attachments are disrupted. In addition, inappropriate alignment and stabilization of osteotomies can lead to disruption of the intraosseous blood supply to the first metatarsal head. Some investigators believe that the addition of a second incision over the first IM space to release the adductor tendon and lateral capsule increases the risk of AVN; however, a low incidence has been reported.[13,15] Potential systemic causes can include the use of tobacco and corticosteroids, metabolic disorders, hemoglobinopathies, and alcoholism.

Symptoms of unresolved pain and swelling may be suggestive of underlying AVN. Following a bunionectomy, radiographic changes to the distal metatarsal characteristic of AVN can be seen; however, not all patients are symptomatic and rarely does it develop into complete AVN of the first metatarsal. The use of bone scans, MRI, bone biopsy, and histopathologic analysis can be used to diagnose AVN. Patients who remain asymptomatic can be managed nonoperatively by immobilizing the hallux with the use of a full-length custom forefoot orthosis with a Morton's extension. When symptoms progress, various surgical options are available, from synovectomy and cheilectomy of the first MTPJ combined with subchondral drilling for mild cases, to resection arthroplasty or MTPJ fusion for severe cases. An interpositional bone graft is typically used to maintain the length of the first ray while adequately removing the avascular bone.

SUMMARY

Surgery for hallux valgus, although technically demanding, has a high rate of success in appropriately selected patients. Relatively few patients have poor outcomes following bunion surgery, but when they do, common diagnostic and treatment dilemmas include recurrent hallux valgus, hallux varus, infection, malunion, and nonunion. Preventing these complications depends on the surgeon's expertise in patient and procedural selection, ability to perform the surgery selected, and knowledge in dealing with postoperative complications.

REFERENCES

1. Coetzee JC, Resig SG, Kuskowski M, et al. The Lapidus procedure as salvage after failed surgical treatment of hallux valgus. Surgical technique. J Bone Joint Surg Am 2004;86(Suppl 1):30–6.
2. Coughlin MJ, Grebing BR, Jones CP. Arthrodesis of the first metatarsophalangeal joint for idiopathic hallux valgus: intermediate results. Foot Ankle Int 2005;26(10): 783–92.
3. Cronin JJ, Limbers JP, Kutty S. Intermetatarsal angle after first metarsaophalangeal joint arthrodesis for hallux valgus. Foot Ankle Int 2006;27(2):104–9.
4. Grimes JS, Coughlin MJ. First metatarsophalangeal joint arthrodesis as a treatment for failed hallux valgus surgery. Foot Ankle Int 2006;27(11):887–93.
5. Horne G, Tanzed T, Ford M. Chevron osteotomy for the treatment of hallux valgus. Clin Orthop Relat Res 1984;183:32–6.

6. Jarde O, Chabaille E, Ganry O, et al. [Recurrent hallux valgus treated with metatarsophalangeal arthrodesis. A series of 32 patients]. Rev Chir Orthop Reparatrice Appar Mot 2001;87(3):257–62 [In French].

7. Kitaoka H, Patzer G. Arthrodesis versus resection arthroplasty for failed hallux valgus operations. Clin Orthop Relat Res 1998;347:208–14.

8. Lagaay PM, Hamilton GA, Ford LA, et al. Rates of revision surgery using Chevron-Austin osteotomy, Lapidus arthrodesis, and closing base wedge osteotomy for correction of hallux valgus deformity. J Foot Ankle Surg 2008;47(4):267–72.

9. Leemrijse T, Hoang B, Maldague P, et al. A new surgical procedure for iatrogenic hallux varus: reverse transfer of the abductor hallucis tendon: a report of 7 cases. Acta Orthop Belg 2008;74(2):227–34.

10. Lehman DE. Salvage of complications of hallux valgus surgery. Foot Ankle Clin 2003;8(1):15–35.

11. Mann RA, Donatto KC. The chevron osteotomy: a clinical and radiographic analysis. Foot Ankle Int 1997;18(5):255–61.

12. Meier PJ, Kenzora JE. The risks and benefits of distal first metatarsal osteotomies. Foot Ankle Int 1985;6(1):7–17.

13. Melillo T. Intraoperative complications of bunion surgery. 2nd edition. New York: Futura Publishing Company; 1991.

14. Rossi WR, Ferreira JC. Chevron osteotomy for hallux valgus. Foot Ankle 1992; 13(7):378–81.

15. Shereff MJ, Yang QM, Kummer FJ. Extraosseous and intraosseous arterial supply to the first metatarsal and metatarsophalangeal joint. Foot Ankle 1987;8(2):81–93.

16. Thomas RL, Espinosa FJ, Richardson EG. Radiographic changes in the first metatarsal head after distal chevron osteotomy combined with lateral release through a plantar approach. Foot Ankle Int 1994;15(6):285–92.

17. Trnka HJ, Zembsch A, Easley ME, et al. The chevron osteotomy for correction of hallux valgus. Comparison of findings after two and five years of follow-up. J Bone Joint Surg Am 2000;82(10):1373–8.

18. Vora AM, Myerson MS. First metatarsal osteotomy nonunion and malunion. Foot Ankle Clin 2005;10(1):35–54.

Current Concepts and Techniques
in Foot and Ankle Surgery

Tibiotalocalcaneal Arthrodesis with the Use of a Humeral Locking Plate

Nicholas J. Lowery, DPM[a], Alison M. Joseph, DPM[a],
Patrick R. Burns, DPM, FACFAS[b],*

KEYWORDS

- Tibiotalocalcaneal arthrodesis • Ankle arthodesis
- Locking plate • Humeral locking plate • Ankle arthritis

Combined arthrosis or deformity of the subtalar and ankle joints presents a challenge to the foot and ankle specialist. Surgical management of this clinical dilemma currently includes combined tibiotalocalcaneal (TTC) arthrodesis, fusion of the subtalar joint with endoprosthesis of the ankle, or joint distraction of the ankle joint with subtalar joint arthrodesis. TTC arthrodesis is a well-described surgical technique that is used for resolution of deformity and end-stage arthrosis of the ankle and subtalar joints and is currently the standard of care for this condition. These conditions can have significant pain and dysfunction and a profound effect on a patient's daily life. Combined rearfoot and ankle disease is seen commonly in posttraumatic arthritis, avascular necrosis of the talus, Charcot neuroarthropathy, and neuromuscular disease.[1–8] Conservative treatment options for these end-stage conditions include the use of anti-inflammatory medications, steroid injections, shoe gear modification, and long-term bracing; however, when these options fail, surgical intervention is indicated.[1–8]

Combined arthrodesis of the subtalar and ankle joints was first described in 1906, and continues to be a powerful option in dealing with complex deformities and revisions.[1] Unfortunately, nonunion rates of 15% and higher have been reported in the literature regarding TTC arthrodesis. A critical factor when performing these types of salvage procedures is achieving stable fixation.[1,3,7–10] Multiple fixation methods have been described in the literature for TTC arthrodesis including screws, blade plates, external fixation, and intramedullary rods.[1–10] Although multiple techniques have been described with varying results, there is no consensus regarding which method of fixation is superior.

[a] University of Pittsburgh Medical Center, South Side Hospital, Pittsburgh, PA, USA
[b] Foot and Ankle Division, Department of Orthopaedic Surgery, University of Pittsburgh Medical Center, South Side Hospital, 2100 Jane Street, Roesch-Taylor Med Bldg North 7100, Pittsburgh, PA 15203, USA
* Corresponding author.
E-mail address: burnsp@upmc.edu (P.R. Burns).

Clin Podiatr Med Surg 26 (2009) 485–492
doi:10.1016/j.cpm.2009.03.011
0891-8422/09/$ – see front matter © 2009 Elsevier Inc. All rights reserved.

podiatric.theclinics.com

A recent trend in orthopedic surgery is the use of locking plate technology, and is the source of much investigation in current literature. Locking plates differ from traditional plates in that they create a fixed-angle single-beam construct, which may increase stability.[11] In conventional configurations, a single screw could fail or become loose, decreasing stability. This traditional configuration relies on adequate bone stock for compression of the plate to bone. In osteopenia or in areas were bicortical fixation is not permitted, this technique is compromised. With locking plate technology, the screws lock to the plate, becoming a single, combined construct making failure less possible. Osteopenia or stress shielding does not lead to screw toggle, loosening, and pull-out. The entire system must fail, which occurs at a much higher force than a single screw. Because of these features, this technology is being applied for use in osteoporotic bone and hard-to-manage fractures where there is limited space for fixation.

Recently, Ahmad and colleagues[1] described the modified use of a proximal humeral locking plate for TTC arthrodesis. The device provided stable fixation by providing internal multiplane stability within the tibia, talus, and calcaneus, and found the plate to be contoured well to the natural anatomy of this area of the lower extremity (**Fig. 1**). Furthermore, the locking design of the plate provided increased stability and rigidity to the surgical site. In their retrospective review, fusion was achieved in 17 (94.4%) of 18 arthrodeses.

The authors have used this technique and find its ease of use and postoperative results advantageous over other methods of fixation. This article highlights the technique of insertion of the humeral locking plate for the stabilization of TTC arthrodesis. A case study is provided to serve as an example of the technique.

INDICATIONS AND CONTRAINDICATIONS

Patients in which TTC arthrodesis is indicated include those with severe degenerative joint disease of the ankle and subtalar joints, deformity, revisional surgery, Charcot

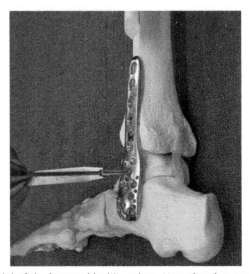

Fig. 1. Saw bone model of the humeral locking plate. Note the plate matches the contour of the lateral foot and ankle without modification.

neuroarthropathy, and instability or progressive neuromuscular disorders that have failed conservative methods.

Unfortunately, the primary cause of ankle and subtalar arthrosis is not wear-and-tear but trauma, most often experienced by the young active population.[12] Typically, patients who are older in age or maintain a sedentary lifestyle tend to have a better prognosis with TTC arthrodesis because the loss of ankle motion is better tolerated in this patient population. Although not contraindicated in the young, active patient special consideration and preoperative consultation and planning must include a frank discussion about the implications of ankle joint fusion and the subsequent loss of motion the patient experiences.

The indications for locking plate fixation include patients who have questionable bone quality or have a history of Charcot neuroarthropathy.[13] Because of the stability of the construct, it is the authors' opinion that these patients are better served with a locking plate versus other common forms of fixation.

Contraindications for TTC arthrodesis include patients unable to be cleared for surgery secondary to medical issues, such as uncontrolled diabetes or poor nutritional status. Peripheral vascular must be evaluated and tobacco use is also a relative contraindication to TTC arthrodesis. When considering internal fixation of any kind, including locking plate fixation, bone infection is also a contraindication and other forms of fixation, specifically external fixation, may be warranted.

PREOPERATIVE PLANNING

As with any operative case, preoperative planning begins with a thorough history and physical examination. The underlying cause of the patient's joint disease must be examined; for example, the posttraumatic patient without deformity but with high functional demand may be treated differently than a patient with severe deformity and bone loss from Charcot neuroarthropathy. A number of etiologic factors can cause hindfoot arthritis, and the root cause must be identified. Included in the history must also be an attempt to discover which conservative measures have been taken by the patient.

Social history is also important. First, patient expectations must be realistic and the discussion must include clinical implications of ankle fusion. Second, the patient must have a support system for postoperative recovery. Finally, the patient should be questioned about the use of tobacco products, because this may affect fusion.

Physical examination is focused on the source of the patient's pain, and examination of both ankle and subtalar range of motion is warranted. Diagnostic injections are also useful in the authors' experience to determine if the pain is caused by subtalar or ankle arthritis. It is important to remember to assess vascular competence; the patient with severe peripheral vascular disease requires adequate work-up with noninvasive or invasive vascular studies. Any presence or history of open wound and infection must be carefully evaluated and the infection and osteomyelitis must be eliminated.

Radiographic evaluation should include standard weightbearing views of the foot and ankle. In addition, calcaneal and long leg axial views are helpful in cases that involve marked deformity and should be evaluated. Advanced imaging, such as CT or MRI, is warranted in specific cases and can be helpful in determining the extent of arthritis or for evaluation of avascular necrosis or osteomyelitis.

OPERATIVE PROCEDURE

The patient is placed in the supine position with a bump under the ipsilateral hip to aid in exposure. A lateral incision is made over the fibula to facilitate a transfibular approach to both joints. The distal fibula is resected and the ankle and subtalar joints are visualized and prepared for fusion.

A 6.5-mm cannulated screw can be placed across the ankle or subtalar joint if necessary to achieve compression, angled from proximal-medial to distal-lateral. The humeral locking plate (Synthes, Paoli, Pennsylvania) is inverted and placed along the lateral aspect of the TTC complex. The plate can be held in place with a drill guide and K-wire. The holes of the plate are filled as necessary. Typically, three to four screws in the tibia, three in the talus, and four to six in the calcaneus are placed depending on anatomy and any loss of height.

Closure is achieved in layers, a drain is placed if desired, and the patient is placed in a compressive dressing and splint.

Tips

The more traditional incision curves anterior as it courses over the subtalar joint. For the current locking plate technique, access to the lateral wall and tuberosity of the calcaneus is required for placement of the plate and screws. The incision for this technique should be continued more linear (**Fig. 2**).

The initial screw placed determines proper placement of the plate. It is placed in the central combination-hole across the dorsal talar dome. If placed too inferior, the next locking screws, just inferior, do not purchase the talus because of their angle (**Fig. 3**).

If necessary, traditional cortical screws may be used in the talar portion of the plate. This is useful with loss of height or deformities where the locking screw angles are not optimal (**Fig. 4**).

The plate allows stable fixation across both joints without screws crossing the joints. This can be useful with implantable bone stimulators. After placement of the stimulator leads, the screws can be placed without worry of damage.

POSTOPERATIVE MANAGEMENT

Patients are admitted and placed in a compression splint immediately following the surgical procedure. The drain, if used, is removed before discharge and sutures are removed between 2 and 3 weeks. The patient is then transitioned into a nonweight-bearing cast until approximately 8 weeks or longer if bony union is not yet complete. Serial radiographs are taken at postoperative visits until bony consolidation is noted. The patient is then transitioned to a walking boot for 1 month. A decision on shoe

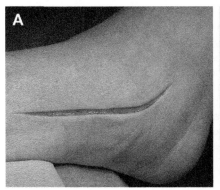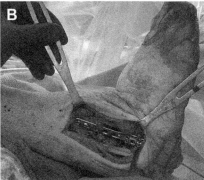

Fig. 2. (A) Standard lateral incision for TTC fusion curving anterior. (B) A more linear modified incision is necessary to accommodate the use of a plate laterally.

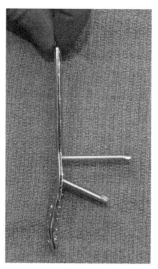

Fig. 3. Side profile of the humeral locking plate showing the orientation of the screws used in talar fixation. Note the angle of the two inferior locking screws. Care should be taken to place these correctly or use traditional cortical screws in these holes to ensure proper fixation.

modifications or the use of a rocker bottom sole is made during the next few months. Patients with abundant midfoot motion may not need these accommodations.

CASE STUDY

A 42-year-old man presented with a chief complaint of right ankle pain for many years duration. He had noticed increasing pain and deformity over the last several months and had sought care from a number of providers. He had tried multiple types of bracing and custom ankle-foot orthosis. As his deformity progressed, he had increasing pain and less ability to ambulate. He did not recall an inciting incident, but had a recent history of instability and continued sprains. His past medical history was significant for asthma; gastroesophageal reflux; obesity; and a history of alcohol abuse, which had led to peripheral neuropathy.

Physical examination of the right lower extremity revealed palpable pulses but absent protective sensation with Semmes-Weinstein monofilament testing. On stance, his right ankle was in a significant varus position with instability. He had pain with attempted range of motion of the right ankle and subtalar joints, and motion was decreased with the knee extended and flexed. Subtalar joint motion was significantly diminished and in maximal eversion, returned to rectus. These deformities were semireducible. Crepitus was noted with attempted right ankle motion. Diagnostic injections provided relief in both the ankle and subtalar joints.

Radiographic examination of the right ankle revealed significant arthritic changes and deformity to both the right ankle and subtalar joints. The anteroposterior view of the ankle showed the ankle joint in varus, and the calcaneal axial view showed the heel in varus. Obvious deformity to the talus and distal tibia was noted from the long-standing deformity.

After failure of conservative care, treatment recommendation to the patient was a TTC arthrodesis to alleviate pain from the end-stage arthrosis of the ankle and

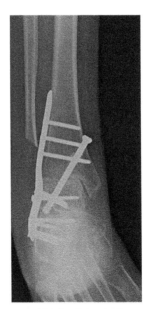

Fig. 4. Example of cortical screws used in the talar component for more optimal position.

subtalar joints and to correct the varus deformity. The choice of fixation was a humeral locking plate modified for the TTC complex. This technique of fixation was used because of the patient's long-standing peripheral neuropathy; the locking fixation would provide added stability to the construct. A bone stimulator was used to augment the primary fusion of this difficult deformity (**Fig. 5**).

DISCUSSION

TTC arthrodesis is a technically challenging surgical procedure used for the treatment of end-stage arthrosis and deformity of the ankle and subtalar joints. Although it is the standard of care for such a condition, there is no consensus concerning the most effective method of fixation. Currently, choices for fixation include blade plates, screws, external fixation, and intramedullary rods and the goal of the procedure is to obtain a solid, pain-free fusion.

Several attempts have been made to discover which method of fixation offers biomechanical superiority. Bennett and colleagues[3] found that three crossed screws may provide more biomechanical stability with regard to micromotion when compared with locked intramedullary nail and two crossed screw configuration. They also compared three crossed screws with an intramedullary construct that was augmented with one bone staple and found that the augmented intramedullary nail allowed less micromotion and provided stability that was almost equal to that of three screws. They postulated that the staple decreased rotational motion, which is inherent to intramedullary constructs. Chiodo and colleagues[13] compared retrograde intramedullary rod with blade plate fixation augmented with a sagittal plane screw and found that the blade plate and screw construct was biomechanically superior, especially in osteopenic bone. Although they point out that blade plate fixation is more technically demanding, they recommend use of blade plate fixation over intramedullary nail in patients with poor bone quality. From these studies, it is suggested that although

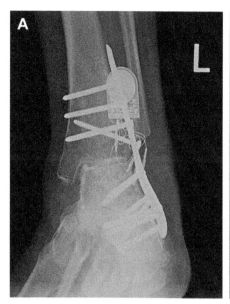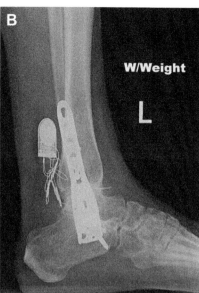

Fig. 5. An oblique (A) and lateral (B) radiograph of the plate used in conjunction with an implantable bone stimulator. This technique allowed for fixation without interfering with the stimulator leads.

retrograde intramedullary nail certainly is an acceptable form of fixation for TTC arthrodesis, other constructs may offer a biomechanical advantage.

Locking plate fixation is a relatively new method of fixation being used in multiple areas of orthopedic surgery. Its advantages include the creation of a fixed angle construct, which increases overall construct stability, and limited contact between the plate and bone, reducing stress on periosteal blood flow.[11] Recently, its use has been applied to TTC arthrodesis.[1]

Chodos and colleagues[4] compared blade plate fixation with the use of a locking plate for TTC arthrodesis. The study design was similar to that of Chiodo and colleagues[13] described previously, and the locking plate used in the study was the Synthes proximal humeral locking plate. The cadaveric study found the locking plate provided higher initial stiffness, higher dorsiflexion and torsional load to failure, and lower construct deformation than blade plate fixation for TTC arthrodesis. They theorize that multiple distal locking screws in diverging planes may provide more stability than the fixed angle blade plate construct, particularly because talar and calcaneal fixation is incorporated. In addition, locking plate fixation may be advantageous not only because of increased stability, but also because it is less technically demanding than blade plate fixation. Furthermore, O'Neill and colleagues[2] found that locking plate fixation had higher final rigidity than intramedullary fixation and conclude that locking plate fixation can be effectively used for TTC arthrodesis.

The use of an inverted humeral locking plate for TTC arthrodesis offers many advantages over other forms of fixation. This particular plate, although designed for the proximal humerus, fits quite well when inverted and applied to the lateral TTC complex. The plate uses locking technology, which offers many biomechanical advantages over conventional plating and other forms of fixation. The screws are also angled in convergent and divergent fashion, which may add to the overall stability of the construct. The technique is not as technically demanding as other forms described, and the plate placed laterally is not prominent when used with a transfibular approach. The authors agree that, in their experience, the proximal humeral locking plate offers excellent biomechanical stability with less technical demand than other forms of fixation.

SUMMARY

The use of a humeral locking plate for TTC arthrodesis is a highly effective form of fixation that offers many biomechanical advantages over other forms of fixation without high technical demand. Use of this plate can also be combined with interfragmentary compression screws across the ankle or subtalar joints or with implantable bone stimulator, as demonstrated in the case example. Its use can be considered when attempting TTC arthrodesis.

REFERENCES

1. Ahmad J, Pour AE, Raikin SM. The modified use of a proximal humeral locking plate for tibiotalocalcaneal arthrodesis. Foot Ankle Int 2007;28(9):977–83.
2. O'Neill PJ, Logel KJ, Parks BG, et al. Rigidity comparison of locking plate and intramedullary fixation for tibiotalocalcaneal arthrodesis. Foot Ankle Int 2008;29(6):581–6.
3. Bennett GL, Cameron B, Njus G, et al. Tibiotalocalcaneal arthrodesis: a biomechanical assessment of stability. Foot Ankle Int 2005;26(7):530–6.
4. Chodos MD, Parks BG, Schon LC, et al. Blade plate compared with locking plate for tibiotalocalcaneal arthrodesis: a cadaver study. Foot Ankle Int 2008;29(2):219–24.
5. Russotti GM, Johnson KA, Cass JR. Tibiotalocalcaneal arthrodesis for arthritis and deformity of the hind part of the foot. J Bone Joint Surg Am 1988;70(9):1304–7.
6. Alfahd U, Roth SE, Stephen D, et al. Biomechanical comparison of intramedullary nail and blade plate fixation for tibiotalocalcaneal arthrodesis. J Orthop Trauma 2005;19(10):703–8.
7. Santangelo JR, Glisson RR, Garras DN, et al. Tibiotalocalcaneal arthrodesis: a biomechanical comparison of multiplanar external fixation with intramedullary fixation. Foot Ankle Int 2008;29(9):936–41.
8. Papa JA, Myerson MS. Pantalar and tibiotalocalcaneal arthrodesis for post-traumatic osteoarthrosis of the ankle and hindfoot. J Bone Joint Surg Am 1992;74:1042–9.
9. Thordarson DB, Markolf K, Cracchiolo A. Stability of an ankle arthrodesis fixed by cancellous-bone screws compared with that fixed by an external fixator. A biomechanical study. J Bone Joint Surg Am 1992;74:1050–5.
10. Easley ME, Montijo HE, Wilson JB, et al. Revision tibiotalar arthrodesis. J Bone Joint Surg Am 2008;90(6):1212–23.
11. Egol KA, Kubiak EN, Fulkerson E, et al. Biomechanics of locked plates and screws. J Orthop Trauma 2004;18(8):488–93.
12. Zgonis T, Stapleton JJ, Roukis TS. Use of circular external fixation for combined subtalar joint fusion and ankle distraction. Clin Podiatr Med Surg 2008;25:745–53.
13. Chiodo CP, Acevedo JI, Sammarco J, et al. Intramedullary rod fixation compared with blade-plate and screw fixation for tibiotalocalcaneal arthrodesis: a biomechanical investigation. J Bone Joint Surg Am 2003;85:2425–38.

Plantar Foot Donor Site as a Harvest of a Split-Thickness Skin Graft

Ronald Belczyk, DPM[a], John J. Stapleton, DPM[b],
Peter A. Blume, DPM, FACFAS[c,d], Thomas Zgonis, DPM, FACFAS[a,*]

KEYWORDS

- Split-thickness skin graft • Diabetic foot ulcers • Plantar foot
- Diabetic wounds • Diabetes mellitus

Soft tissue reconstruction of the glabrous skin on the plantar and digital surfaces in patients with diabetes mellitus can be a challenge to the reconstructive surgeon. Although, there are many treatment options available, such as local wound care, bioengineered alternative tissues, split- and full-thickness skin grafts, local random flaps, and muscle and pedicle flaps, defects of the sole or digit require soft tissue coverage that can withstand maximal pressure and shear forces encountered during ambulation.[1] When feasible, local random flaps are advantageous and are a good option for providing soft tissue coverage for these wounds. Often, wounds to the digits are not amenable to soft tissue coverage, and affected digits are likely to be amputated because of exposed deep structures like bone, tendon, or joint capsule that become easily exposed once skin breakdown occurs. Pinch grafts from the sinus tarsi, popliteal crease, or groin offer the surgeon the ability to harvest a full-thickness skin graft (FTSG) that can provide durable coverage if the graft survives. Unfortunately, in the diabetic patient with vascular compromise, these grafts are likely to fail. In addition, they create full-thickness skin defects at the donor site that require primary closure. Closure of these donor sites is easily accomplished among healthy patients but is associated with more difficulty in the diabetic population with long-standing venous insufficiency or lymphedema.

Split-thickness skin grafts (STSGs) in the diabetic foot offer many advantages.[2] STSGs are easy to perform; offer a better chance of survival as compared with

[a] Division of Podiatric Medicine and Surgery, Department of Orthopaedic Surgery, The University of Texas Health Science Center at San Antonio, San Antonio, TX, USA
[b] Foot and Ankle Surgery, VSAS Orthopaedics, Allentown, PA, USA
[c] Department of Orthopaedics and Rehabilitation, Yale School of Medicine, New Haven, CT, USA
[d] North American Center for Limb Preservation, New Haven, CT, USA
* Corresponding author.
E-mail address: zgonis@uthscsa.edu (T. Zgonis).

Clin Podiatr Med Surg 26 (2009) 493–497
doi:10.1016/j.cpm.2009.04.003
0891-8422/09/$ – see front matter © 2009 Elsevier Inc. All rights reserved.

FTSGs, especially in vascularly compromised patients; and are usually associated with little morbidity at the donor site. STSGs are cost-effective and can be repeated if needed.[1–5]

A basic principle in soft tissue reconstruction of the diabetic foot is to cover "the lost tissue" with "like tissue."[2,5–11] In general, skin varies from body site to body site. Skin from the eyelid, postauricular and supraclavicular areas, medial thigh, and upper extremity is thin, whereas skin from the back, buttocks, palms of the hands, and soles of the feet is much thicker. Plastic surgeons have found this principle useful when reconstructing glabrous soft tissue defects of the volar aspect of the hand after lengthening procedures for postburn contractures.[11]

Roukis[8] reported a novel technique of harvesting a STSG from the medial longitudinal arch of the foot to avoid donor site complications by harvesting the graft from the weight-bearing aspect of the foot. The authors have also found that this technique provides durable skin coverage almost comparable to a FTSG. Some inherent difficulties with this technique were encountered, however, particularly the ability to obtain a symmetric graft from the irregular and limited surface area of the medial longitudinal arch. Often, the harvested skin grafts would display irregular borders and were asymmetric. In addition, harvesting from this area was difficult secondary to the prominent medial band of the plantar fascia and the bone prominences of the medial column, which would limit the placement and orientation of the dermatome while harvesting the graft. For these reasons, the authors have altered this novel technique by harvesting durable plantar skin with inherent characteristics that can withstand weight-bearing forces to selected soft tissue defects and non–weight-bearing surfaces. In this article, we present a case report in which a STSG was harvested directly from the plantar aspect of the foot to cover an ulceration located on the medial aspect of the ipsilateral foot and previous partial first ray amputation. No observed complications were noted from the donor or recipient site.

SURGICAL TECHNIQUE

After patient education and medical optimization, the wound is adequately debrided and converted from a contaminated or infected wound into a clean wound. Intraoperative cultures along with clinical presentation usually determine the need and length of antibiotic therapy. A thorough vascular assessment is performed, and vascular intervention is initiated if necessary. The following are descriptions in greater depth of how the authors approach these soft tissue defects and the technique of harvesting the STSG from the plantar aspect of the foot.

The recipient bed is prepared by debriding all necrotic, infected, fibrotic, or avascular tissue. It is important to ensure that the wound bed is well vascularized and all nonviable and infected tissue has been excised before performing this procedure.[2,7,12] Granulation tissue is an indicator of skin graft readiness and survival. Absence of granulation tissue may be secondary to ischemia, contamination, or infection. If ischemia is present, further vascular imaging and intervention may be needed. Definitive soft tissue coverage should be delayed until arterial perfusion is sufficient for wound healing.

When dealing with chronic ulcers, the surgeon needs to ensure that active infection is not present. The authors recommend ulcer debridement in the operating room, wherein deep soft tissue cultures are obtained. In addition, bone cultures are taken if osteomyelitis is suspected. Once antibiotics are initiated, the wound is then clinically assessed to determine the need for staged soft tissue coverage procedures. A decision for skin grafting is based on the clinical appearance of the wound while the patient is placed on antibiotics for the infection. Deep infection involving bone may be managed with bone resection and long-term antibiotics based on intraoperative cultures. Unfortunately, in most cases, when dealing with digital ulcers and underlying osteomyelitis, an amputation is preferred rather than soft tissue coverage after debridement. Wounds that are amenable to skin grafting are further prepared by hydrosurgery techniques, which offer a unique advantage in removing minimal amounts of tissue while simultaneously irrigating the wound to prevent bacterial contamination.

After preparing the wound or recipient bed, one would begin harvesting the plantar STSG with a power dermatome. Typically, when a plantar STSG is harvested, it is to provide soft tissue coverage of a small wound. Usually, a 1-in dermatome set at twenty one thousandths of an inch is sufficient. The surgeon holds the dermatome at approximately 45° to the skin and applies firm and constant pressure while advancing the dermatome from the direction of the toes toward the heel. Harvesting the graft in this direction prevents crossing the thick glabrous skin while allowing the surgical assistant easy access to obtain the graft from the dermatome as it is harvested.

Surgeons may harvest a STSG slightly smaller than the recipient site to obtain the appropriate size to cover the wound because meshing of the graft increases its surface area. The STSG can be meshed up to a ratio of 1:1.5. Meshing the graft permits drainage of fluid from beneath the graft, which helps to prevent seroma, hematoma, and infection.

The harvested STSG can be augmented with platelet-rich plasma and then secured to the wound bed with nonabsorbent sutures of low reactivity or skin staples. The excess skin can be excised, and a bolster dressing is then applied based on the surgeon's preference. The patient is immobilized with a splint, cast, or external fixation device for an average of 4 to 6 weeks. In the authors' experience, the bolster dressing can be removed approximately 14 to 21 days after the surgical procedure. At that point, the patient is progressed to protective weight bearing and is ultimately transitioned to custom-molded or extra-depth shoes with double inserts to avoid future ulceration. Negative pressure wound therapy can also be applied to the recipient STSG area and is usually left uninterrupted for 5 to 7 days (**Fig. 1**).

DISCUSSION

Glabrous skin grafting has been applied widely for coverage of smaller defects in the hand and foot and has yielded superior results with improved function, sensation, appearance, and durability.[8–11,13] The concept of reconstructing plantar defects by this method has probably been impeded by the broadly held belief that the donor site would have significant complications, such as excessive scarring, pain, and functional deficit. This technique varies from prior technique descriptions because the donor site is from the plantar surface of the foot. The authors' patient showed reliable and durable results, with excellent tissue coverage and no contracture. In addition, this technique is easy to perform and can be considered for soft tissue defects of the digits or plantar surfaces that are amenable to a STSG and cannot be closed through other more traditional techniques.

Ultimately, this is another option to consider for soft tissue reconstruction of diabetic foot wounds to help restore form and function and to prevent amputation. The authors do not recommend this technique for all soft tissue wounds of the toes and plantar aspect of the foot but believe it is a viable option for selected small diabetic foot wounds that may benefit from a STSG. In conclusion, the authors

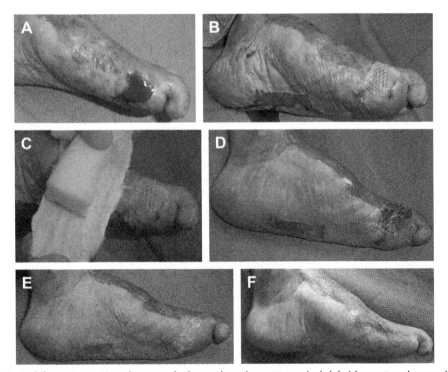

Fig.1. (*A*) Intraoperative photograph shows the adequate surgical debridement and wound bed preparation at the recipient site. The patient presented with a chronic open wound at the partial first ray amputation site and a history of diabetes mellitus and peripheral neuropathy. (*B*) Intraoperative photograph shows the donor site from the plantar surface of the foot and application to the recipient site. (*C*) STSG was then stapled to the recipient site and secured with a bolster dressing consisting of nonadherent gauze and a sterile sponge soaked in saline. (*D*) Postoperative clinical appearance of the donor and recipient sites at 3 weeks and after removal of the bolster dressing. Clinical photographs at 6 weeks (*E*) and 6 months (*F*) after surgery.

present a minimally invasive procedure for harvesting a STSG from the plantar surface of the foot.

REFERENCES

1. Levin L. The reconstructive ladder: an orthoplastic approach. Orthop Clin North Am 1993;24:393–409.
2. Zgonis T, Stapleton JJ, Roukis TS. Advanced plastic surgery techniques for soft tissue coverage of the diabetic foot. Clin Podiatr Med Surg 2007;24(3):547–68, x.
3. Ratner D. Skin grafting: from here to there. Dermatol Clin 1998;16:75–90.
4. Ablove R, Howell R. The physiology and technique of skin grafting. Hand Clin 1997;13:163–73.
5. Jolly GP, Zgonis T, Blume P. Soft tissue reconstruction of the diabetic foot. Clin Podiatr Med Surg 2003;20(4):757–81.
6. Roukis TS, Zgonis T. Skin grafting techniques for soft-tissue coverage of diabetic foot and ankle wounds. J Wound Care 2005;14(4):173–6.

7. Zgonis T, Stapleton JJ, Rodriguez RH, et al. Plastic surgery reconstruction of the diabetic foot. AORN J 2008;87(5):951–66, quiz 967–70.
8. Roukis TS. Use of the medial arch as a donor site for split-thickness skin grafts. J Foot Ankle Surg 2003;42(5):312–4.
9. Grumbine N. Split-thickness skin grafts from the junctional skin of the arch. Clin Podiatr Med Surg 1986;3(2):259–67.
10. Banis J. Glabrous skin grafts for plantar defects. Foot Ankle Clin 2001;6(4): 827–37.
11. Simman R. Medial plantar arch pinch grafts are an effective technique to resurface palmar and plantar wounds. Ann Plast Surg 2004;53(3):256–60.
12. Zgonis T, Stapleton JJ, Jeffries LC, et al. Surgical treatment of Charcot neuropathy. AORN J 2008;87(5):971–86, quiz 987–90.
13. Sams H, McDonald M, Stasko T. Useful adjuncts to harvest split-thickness skin grafts. Dermatol Surg 2004;30:1591–2.

Index

Note: Page numbers of article titles are in **boldface** type.

Clin Podiatr Med Surg 26 (2009) 499–505
doi:10.1016/S0891-8422(09)00048-2
0891-8422/09/$ – see front matter © 2009 Elsevier Inc. All rights reserved.

podiatric.theclinics.com

Moving?

Make sure your subscription moves with you!

To notify us of your new address, find your **Clinics Account Number** (located on your mailing label above your name), and contact customer service at:

E-mail: elspcs@elsevier.com

800-654-2452 (subscribers in the U.S. & Canada)
314-453-7041 (subscribers outside of the U.S. & Canada)

Fax number: 314-523-5170

Elsevier Periodicals Customer Service
11830 Westline Industrial Drive
St. Louis, MO 63146

*To ensure uninterrupted delivery of your subscription, please notify us at least 4 weeks in advance of move.

ELSEVIER

Printed and bound by CPI Group (UK) Ltd, Croydon, CR0 4YY

03/10/2024

01040465-0016